Surviving the "Flesh-Eating Bacteria"

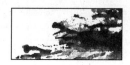

Surviving the "Flesh-Eating Bacteria"

Understanding, Preventing, Treating, and Living with the Effects of Necrotizing Fasciitis

Jacqueline A. Roemmele

and

Donna Batdorff

AVERY

a member of

Penguin Putnam Inc.

New York

Most Avery books are available at special quantity discounts for bulk purchase for sales promotions, premiums, fund-raising, and educational needs. Special books or book excerpts also can be created to fit specific needs. For details, write Putnam Special Markets, 375 Hudson Street, New York, NY 10014.

Proceeds from the publication of this book will benefit the National Necrotizing Fasciitis Foundation.

The illustration on page 4 was reprinted with permission from Thomas A. Raffin, M.D.

a member of
Penguin Putnam Inc.
375 Hudson Street
New York, NY 10014
www.penguinputnam.com

Library of Congress Catologing-in-Publication Data

Roemmele, Jacqueline A.
Surviving the "flesh-eating bacteria": understanding, preventing, treating, and living with
the effects of necrotizing fasciitis / Jacqueline A. Roemmele & Donna Batdorff.
p. cm.
Includes bibliographical references and index.
ISBN 1-58333-071-2
1. Necrotizing fasciitis—Popular works. I. Batdorff, Donna. II. Title.
RC116.S84 R64   2000   00-042106
616.9'2—dc21

Printed in the United States of America
1   3   5   7   9   10   8   6   4   2

Book design by Tanya Maiboroda

To my children, Vincent, Alex, and Ricardo, with oceans of love.
Mom's going to be just fine now.

—JACQUELINE ROEMMELE

To Linda Troyer, my friend, who made sure I got to the hospital;
Judy Steortz, my sister, who made sure I survived; and Kevin
Reynolds, my friend, who gives me ongoing encouragement.

—DONNA BATDORFF

The authors dedicate this book also to all those who have survived
necrotizing fasciitis and to those who have lost their lives to
necrotizing fasciitis. Let it not be in vain.

Contents

✿

Part Three: Life After NF

Acknowledgments

꩜

THIS BOOK could not have been possible without the wealth of information freely contributed to us from hundreds of people all over the world. Our warmest thanks to you all, including Bob Borge, Mary Burge, Cindy Charlton, David Cowles, Grant Drummond, Paul Fasolas, Doug Fitzpatrick, Rose and Betty Goude, Lee Graybiel, Sheri Hardin, Maureen Heath, Ray Holst, Katie Lambert, Theresa Lee, Mary Catherine Habeck-Leighou, Carole Manley, Scott Miller, Cassi Moore, Ann Perry, Carol Rolfe, Bo Salisbury, Stephanie Sebastian, Cindy Weitzel, and many, many others.

Also our heartfelt gratitude to the families of the following individuals who lost their lives to NF: Pamela Berkemeir, Mathew Cahill, Susan Dougherty, Diana Ferguson, Dave Firth, Jeanne Herrington, Joseph Magliocco, Earvin A. Mayfield, Jr., Rebekah McVay, Arnold Robertson, Hailey Elizabeth Stone, and so many others.

We would also like to offer our sincerest appreciation to the following medical professionals who gave freely and generously of their time and energy to contribute their expertise, and/or to review our manuscript to ensure that it reflected the reality of NF: Drs. Alan Bisno, Alfred Bollet, Alan Cohen, Ralph Costanzo, James Dale, Jay Early, Vincent Fischetti, Tamara Fishman, Dennis Hammond, Laurence Hollands, Anthony Holler, Donald Low, James Majeski, Christopher McHenry, James Oliver, Dennis Stevens, Steven Triesenberg; Robert Weinstein, Irene Koenig; Deborah Mitnick, LCSW-C; Carolyn West, RN; and Carol Wallace, CRC.

We are both also deeply grateful to Avery/Penguin Putnam for realizing the tremendous need for this book, and to our editor, Dara Stewart, for her excellent work on our behalf. Many thanks as well to Kristen Forbes for cheerfully keeping us organized and sane. We would also like to acknowledge the incredible power of the Internet. Without it, we would not have met. Without it, necrotizing fasciitis would still be an unknown, rarely heard about condition. The "Net" has allowed us to inform more than 125,000 people about necrotizing fasciitis through our Web site, www.nnff.org.

❀

There are so many people throughout my life that I would like to recognize for their inspiration, encouragement, love, hard-earned lessons, friendship, and unwavering support. To my mom, Jacqui Roemmele, whom I believe probably saved my life with her sixth sense and stubbornness, and my dad, Vincent J. Roemmele, who taught me to be strong in the face of any adversity, I love you both! To Rick Sanchez, father of my amazing children, all my love for being there for me through it all—from changing my dressings while I was sick, to comforting me through the darkest hours, to telling me I was still beautiful no matter what I saw in the mirror. To my brilliant son Vincent, for teaching me so many lessons about perseverance and integrity. To my son Alex "Seinfeld" for the laughter when I was at my wits' end, and to my son Ricky for quietly slipping me a fresh cup of coffee or iced tea as I stared at the computer screen writing this book. Thank you, boys, for your patience and understanding while I was dedicated to this important project. I hope it makes you proud one day. To Roberto, Ebe, and Norma Sanchez, for your many gifts to me. *Te quiero mucho.* Lots of love to my brothers, Tom and Richard Roemmele, as well. Friends and family I hold close in my heart—the late Russell Roemmele, mentor and uncle who encouraged my writing ever since I was a little girl; Monte, Laurie, and my miracle godson Mychael Roberts; Joe and Lucille Giordano, Joanne Johnson, Noreen O'Keeffe, Linda Sullivan, Eileen Miller, Michelle Bergeron, Carol Georgacopoulos, Carlos Hernandez-Chavez, Michelle Salvatore-Porrino, Valerie Wampler, Dave Lobeck, Bruce Motta, and Kevin McGarry. My warmest thanks also to Nick Magnapera for your encouragement and faith in me. To P.D., as well, my very dear friend, for the gift of wings, and the courage to trust them. My warmest thanks also to John Pagnozzi, M.D.; Clifford Stirba, M.D.; Donald McIntyre, Ph.D.; Hubert Weinberg, M.D.; Jacques Parenteau, Esq.; Kathleen Coleman, Esq.; Frank Bailey, Esq.; and John Rowley, Esq.

—Jacqueline Roemmele

⑥

First I want to thank my wonderful friend and coauthor, Jacqueline Roemmele. This book was her passion, and the bulk of it is her doing. My goal to inform others about necrotizing fasciitis came about as a result of my miracle story of survival. I believe I survived necrotizing fasciitis due, in large part, to the prayers of many people I knew and people I did not know. I thank God for listening to these prayers. Leading this group was my sister Judy. Friends who were there to encourage me were Kevin Reynolds, Jim Miars, Scott Swanson, Linda Troyer, Amy Miller, Sandy VanderZicht, Anna Moore Butzner, Mary Kay Parks, Nancy Benner, Cathy Amodeo, Cherri Alberts, Lafayette Beers, Tom Soltys, Joe Crump, Sue Owens, Valerie Cutler Walker, Linda Voss-Graham, and Brian Borbot. Sandy also provided literary guidance, as did Barbara D'Amato and Stan Gundry. Last but certainly not least, I wish to acknowledge my deceased parents, Jim and Opal, who taught me the skills of survival and determination to handle all that life hands out.

—Donna Batdorff

Foreword

✦

NECROTIZING fasciitis (NF) is a severe and progressive infection of the tissues situated between the skin and underlying muscle. As the process spreads along tissue planes, blood supply is lost and gangrene ensues, leading to loss of limbs or, all too frequently, to death. A particularly vicious form of NF is that caused by the group A streptococcus, the same bacterium responsible for common "strep throat" and scarlet fever. Because of the highly destructive and rapidly progressive nature of streptococcal NF, the organism has been dubbed in the lay press as the "flesh-eating bug."

NF due to the group A streptococcus is not a new disease. Descriptions of what was more than likely streptococcal NF are found in the writings of Hippocrates (circa 400 B.C.), and the disease was first reported in the modern medical literature by Dr. Frank Meleney in 1924. In the intervening years, however, such cases have been extremely rare. Indeed, until a decade ago, neither I, a physician specializing for many years in infectious diseases and with an investigative interest in the group A streptococcus, nor my colleagues had more than a rare encounter with cases of "flesh-eating disease." Since that time, however, and for reasons not yet entirely understood, the incidence of group A streptococcal NF has increased both in the United States and abroad, and clusters of the disease have appeared in many communities. Moreover, strep NF is often accompanied by a toxic shock syndrome similar to the tampon-associated shock syndrome caused by staphylococcus. Unfortunately, when NF is accompanied by toxic shock, the mortality rate ranges between 30 and 70 percent.

Although the risk of strep NF and toxic shock is highest at the extremes of life and in patients with certain chronic diseases, the disease may also strike perfectly normal individuals who may progress from good health to death's door in only a few days. Such cases occur unpredictably, and there is no way of preventing them. Thus this disease understandably strikes fear in family members and associates of stricken patients as well as in communities where it is occurring in increased numbers. In such circumstances, people search for information and for comfort and reassurance from persons who have suffered from the illness and survived.

As survivors, Jacqueline and Donna have devoted themselves to disseminating information about the so-called flesh-eating disease by cofounding the National Necrotizing Fasciitis Foundation and establishing a Web site that serves as an information resource and support group for victims and family members. By involving authoritative medical experts, the foundation has dispelled rumor and misinformation and served as a valuable data collection center for researchers studying strep NF. Through this forum, it has been possible to inform the public that strep NF remains a rare disease and that, promptly recognized and treated, the chances of survival are greatly improved.

This book serves as a valuable distillation of information for those who have experienced strep NF themselves or in loved ones, as well as for the general public. It is written with a minimum of the technical jargon we doctors often use (and overuse!), so the message is readily understandable to the nonprofessional. The true-life case histories are heart wrenching, often sad, and sometimes inspiring.

The earliest symptoms of strep NF often simulate other and much more common illnesses. Diagnosis can thus be difficult, even for experienced physicians. In addition, some physicians may not yet be entirely familiar with the illness, which is still quite uncommon in everyday medical practice. Thus, it is important for the lay public to recognize the warning signs that should alert them to seek medical advice, to question their physicians about the possibility of NF, and if necessary, to seek second opinions from qualified infectious disease specialists. This information is lucidly presented in the following pages. Finally, the reader will be glad to know about encouraging research into prevention of NF and other group A streptococcal diseases by development of a safe and effective vaccine.

Let's hope that a future second edition of this book will be able to detail great progress in diagnosis and treatment of the "flesh-eating disease" or even a vaccine to make it largely of historic interest.

—Alan L. Bisno, M.D.
Chief, Medical Service
Miami Veterans Affairs Medical Center
Professor and Vice-Chairman
University of Miami School of Medicine

Preface

❦

My EXPERIENCE with necrotizing fascitiis and the fallout that followed was without question the most painful time of my life—physically, mentally, emotionally, and spiritually. The disease ravaged my body and left me disfigured and scarred. But like so many survivors of a traumatic event, I have since developed a profound sense of purpose and psychic freedom in my life. I've changed for the better. I find that I am no longer tethered to petty or superficial illusions about myself or others. Once as vain as a Siamese cat, today you're more likely to find me makeup-free and barefoot in the garden with my hair in a ponytail. Once an aggressive businesswoman who put my children second to chase an elusive, dazzling career, after my illness I realized that life—and my three little boys—were far too precious. Finding myself fed up one day, I packed a box of my belongings, took one last look around my lovely office, squeezed my eyes closed, and made the irreversible decision to leap off the corporate roller coaster that had controlled my life for far too long. To my surprise, I landed on soft ground—a cushion of inner peace, clarity, and courage hard earned like so many other people in this world by triumphing over one of life's unexpected tragedies. I then started my own Web site development and marketing business from my home, where I can be a full-time mom as well. I love every moment of it.

But this did not happen right away. After my wounds healed, I struggled through all of the classic stages of grieving compounded a thousand times by my decision to file suit against the physician who I believe failed to recognize my infection. I was severely depressed, gained sixty pounds, and was plagued by an irrational fear that kept me semi-confined to my house for many months. I alienated myself from my friends and shunned contact with other people. My children saw only a shadow of the mother they knew and loved. My husband, Rick, ran out of ideas to try to help me, although he never wavered in his loyalty and affection.

So as a matter of survival, in late 1996, I attempted to reach out to someone who had experienced what I had. I searched the Internet and eventually stumbled onto the Web site of Donna Batdorff, another survivor of necrotizing fasciitis. I e-mailed her, and with her warm and friendly response, the course of my life was forever altered. Donna and I forged a strong and empowering friendship, bonded by our unique battles against this microscopic killer. We realized that we were destined to meet and to join forces to do what we could to fill the void of information and to offer support for other victims and their families. So, together, in early 1997, Donna and I founded the National Necrotizing Fasciitis Foundation (NNFF). What has since evolved for us and the foundation has been truly inspiring and humbling. Thousands of people from all walks of life, from all over the world, have reached out to us when NF invades their lives. We are the leading source of information available about NF, and have brought together hundreds of people who find kinship, support, and comfort in each other. Both Donna and I are very proud to be fulfilling the foundation's mission to make a difference in the understanding, awareness, diagnosis, and treatment of necrotizing fasciitis. This book is the natural evolution of this mission.

Through the publication of this book, we hope that we can accomplish three critical goals: to provide a comprehensive resource about necrotizing fasciitis for victims of NF and their loved ones that will answer all of their lingering questions regarding what they went through and why; to greatly reduce the number of missed and/or delayed diagnoses that occur by educating doctors and nurses about the symptoms, manifestations, and treatment of NF; and to teach the general public, from children to the elderly, prevention techniques, how to recognize the symptoms of NF, and how to talk to their doctors so that future cases of NF can be avoided or significantly minimized.

I know that at this moment there are many survivors of NF in the world who feel the way I did—depressed, confused, and mourning the loss of physical beauty, range of motion, limbs, and their previous lifestyle. We truly hope that you will discover a seed of inspiration in this book to carry you through your personal grieving process. For the parents, children, siblings, husbands, and wives of those who lost the battle against necrotizing fasciitis, we pray that you find peace and healing through finally understanding this devastating disease.

—Jacqueline A. Roemmele

Author's Note

⑥

THROUGHOUT this book, the authors share the personal accounts of many people affected by NF. Many of these accounts were shared with us through the contributor's public posting on our Web site, www.nnff.org. In some cases, we have changed the name of the individual and his or her identifying characteristics to protect his or her privacy.

PART ONE

⑥

All About Necrotizing Fasciitis

"Hello, my name is John, and I am a survivor of necromantic fasculitis, or whatever it's called. . . ."

"Necrotizing fasciitis? Oh, I've heard of that— it's like Ebola, right? How the heck did you catch that here in the United States?"

"The flesh-eating bacteria is proof that the world is coming to an end. Better get ready."

"I've heard it's caused by a spider bite."

NECROTIZING fasciitis is one of the most misunderstood diseases of our time. Because of the lack of information available to the general public regarding its origin, its cause, and who is at risk, rumors and half-truths have persisted. Coupling this with shocking headlines of swift, horrible deaths and reported outbreaks, the disease has become the stuff of nightmares. Part One of this book will set the record straight once and for all about necrotizing fasciitis. It will detail the infection's history, what causes it, how it attacks, and who is at greater risk of contracting it.

⑥

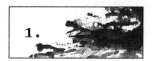

1.

What Is Necrotizing Fasciitis?

NECROTIZING FASCIITIS (pronounced NECK-roe-tie-zing FASH-ee-EYE-tis) means "decaying infection of the fascia," the sheets of connective tissue surrounding the muscles. This sudden and vicious infection is caused by one or more kinds of bacteria, which the media has nicknamed "the flesh-eating bacteria," that attack the skin, the fat of the subcutaneous tissue (the tissue located just beneath the skin), and fasciae, causing the affected areas to necrose, or die. (See Figure 1.1 on page 4 for a depiction of the layers of soft tissue of the body.) Gangrene, toxemia (poisons from the bacteria traveling throughout the body), organ failure, and death are often the result. It is caused by multiple bacteria, that act synergistically to produce a rapidly progressive infection. Less commonly, necrotizing fasciitis can be caused by toxins produced by a single organism, like invasive group A streptococcus.

Necrotizing fasciitis, or NF, as we will refer to it throughout this book, most often enters the body through a weakness or break in the skin and spreads very quickly—sometimes inches an hour (hence the illusion of being "flesh-eating"). Although NF can strike any part of the body, the most common areas are the extremities, the abdominal wall, and the perineum (the area encompassing the anus and genitalia). It will kill the victim if not aggressively treated within a short time after the ini-

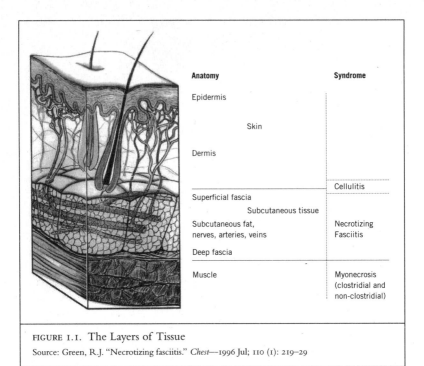

FIGURE I.I. The Layers of Tissue

Source: Green, R.J. "Necrotizing fasciitis." *Chest*—1996 Jul; 110 (1): 219–29

tial symptoms present. Even with treatment, the disease kills as many as three out of ten victims. The earlier the patient receives proper medical care, the better the chances are for survival. Repeated surgeries to cut away infected tissue, including amputation of fingers, toes, and limbs; intravenous antibiotic therapy; and nutritional support may be required to save the life of the patient. If the victim has succumbed to toxic shock— an often fatal occurrence in patients suffering from NF that causes systemic organ failure—hemodialysis, induced sedation, additional drugs, endotracheal intubation (a technique used to keep the airways of critically ill patients clear), and various high-powered drugs may also be required. Depending upon the type of bacteria involved in the infection, hyperbaric (high-pressure) oxygen treatments may also be utilized. Lengthy periods of recovery and rehabilitation are often required, including daily dressing changes and skin grafting to cover gaping wounds. Patients are often left with a mutilated appearance, with large "shark-bite–looking" contours and scars. The psychological and emotional impact on the victims and their families can be devastating.

Symptoms of Necrotizing Fasciitis

Each case of necrotizing fasciitis follows a unique course that is influenced by many variables, such as the type of bacteria involved, the patient's health status before infection, and the area of the body attacked. The course of the disease, severity of symptoms, and speed of progression of the disease will also vary from person to person. With that said, following is the general classic progression of symptoms of NF.

Early Symptoms

Early symptoms of NF usually occur one to five days after contracting the bacteria. They begin with symptoms that are often mistaken for the flu. These include high fever, sore throat, stomachache, nausea, diarrhea, chills, general body aches, and malaise (a general feeling of being unwell). Around the same time, the patient notices soreness in a limb or particular area of the body, such as the upper arm, abdomen, inner thigh, ankle, or foot. Very often, a cut, scratch, bruise, or boil may be noticed in the general area of the soreness. The patient commonly thinks, "I must have injured myself when I was playing/gardening/moving boxes/skiing."

Unfortunately, early symptoms of NF are often brushed off as being related to an underlying illness, flu, or postoperative symptoms, which results in a tragic delay in diagnosis. The infection is then allowed to advance.

Advanced Symptoms

Usually only a day or two after the onset of early symptoms, the flulike symptoms continue to worsen, resulting in cycles of diarrhea and vomiting. Fever can reach and even surpass 104°F. The limb pain progresses from being occasional and annoying to constant and piercing. A portion of the limb or affected area may appear bright red, shiny, swollen, and very hot to the touch. The patient will feel dehydrated, with infrequent urination or none at all. As symptoms progress, the affected area continues to swell and becomes purple or mottled (blotches of black, purple, and red) in appearance, and a rash of blisters may appear. The rash then begins to spread to adjoining areas of the body. The affected limb may feel almost wooden when palpated. The pain becomes excruciating. The patient may have extremely low blood pressure (hypotension) and a faint, rapid heartbeat (tachycardia), which causes dizziness, weakness, and confusion. The skin may take on the texture of an orange peel.

Critical Symptoms

About one to three days after the advanced symptoms begin, the patient's confusion and weakness become pronounced. He or she may repeatedly lose consciousness. The affected area swells to several times the normal size and may split open, discharging large amounts of thin, cloudy drainage fluid resembling dishwater. Large blisters (called bullae) filled with a bloody or a yellowish fluid appear on the affected limb. Blackened necrotic lesions appear, causing the skin to break open. The pain, which had been unbearable, gives way to anesthesia (lack of sensation) as nerves are destroyed. Urine output ceases completely (a condition called anuria). Blood pressure drops severely and may become imperceptible, heartbeat is rapid and shallow (tachycardia), breathing becomes rapid (tachypnea), and the patient becomes delirious. The patient's vital internal organs, such as the kidneys, liver, and lungs, shut down due to toxic shock. The skin and other tissues can become blackened and slough off the body. Death follows shortly.

Incidence of Necrotizing Fasciitis

Necrotizing fasciitis does not favor one culture, geographical location, or gender. Some people with pre-existing illnesses and conditions are at higher risk, although anyone—from the newborn to the elderly—can become infected.

Most estimates suggest that there are between one and five cases of NF per 100,000 people per year. However, as we'll explain, the actual number of cases in the United States and abroad at any given time is difficult to approximate. Leading researchers do agree, however, that while NF is a relatively rare disease, the incidence of infection is on the rise. This is especially true in developing countries. In fact, the Centers for Disease Control (CDC) consider invasive group A streptococcus (a major cause of NF) to be an important concern. The Centers have spearheaded a special program called the Active Bacterial Core Surveillance Emerging Infections Program Network to monitor cases of illness caused by this bacterium in California, Connecticut, Georgia, Maryland, Minnesota, New York, and Oregon—a population of over 17.5 million people.

In Canada, researchers at Mt. Sinai Hospital in Toronto, Ontario, have been actively tracking invasive group A strep incidence since 1992 in a population of over 11.4 million people. (See the Resources section of this book for more information regarding these two surveillance studies). And yet, these worthwhile programs still do not paint a complete picture of the number of people affected by NF. This is largely due to the fact that NF is often caused by a handful of other types of bacteria in addition to invasive group A strep, and these cases are not factored into the statistical data.

Other researchers have argued that the number of NF cases has not substantially increased over the years but that more cases have come to the public's attention because of increased media attention. This is an interesting point, but while we recognize the media's avid interest in NF, we do not agree that publicity is the root of the apparent surge in cases. According to the medical literature, as well as our own experience, unquestionably there are more cases of NF now than in prior decades. In addition, as awareness grows, more cases are being properly diagnosed. Moreover, while NF is reported often in the press, we receive hundreds of reports from NF victims and their families that have never made the headlines.

Clusters of Invasive Group A Strep Infections

In recent years, several clusters or mini-outbreaks of invasive group A strep have made national headlines. One such outbreak occurred in Texas during the early months of 1998. Over 250 cases of invasive group A strep were reported, resulting in over forty deaths, including a number of children. Over sixty children, some with chickenpox, developed invasive infections as well.

As another example, in late February and early March of 1999, a cluster of invasive group A strep infections was reported in the Chicago area, causing over a dozen deaths. Researchers studying the phenomenon do not have a clear answer as to the cause of geographically isolated clusters of invasive group A infections. What is known, however, is the following:

- The onset of the clusters seems to coincide with the expected time of year (winter, spring) for strep throat infections.
- While many people within the area may contract strep throat, which is contagious, few will fall victim to invasive infections like necrotizing fasciitis and streptococcal toxic shock syndrome.
- Those that do fall victim to the invasive group A strep infections are typically at higher risk to begin with, such as the elderly, chronically ill, and children with chickenpox.

Some researchers theorize that a particularly virulent strain of group A strep causes mini-outbreaks, although studies have shown that strains of bacteria cultured from victims within the same cluster have not been identical.

Survival Rate and What Affects It

The mortality rate for NF can be anywhere from 30 to 80 percent. Without medical treatment, death from NF is certain; however, the survival rate, as well as the degree of amputation and/or debridement of flesh necessary, does improve dramatically the earlier the infection is properly diagnosed and treated. The patient's chance for survival is better if the diagnosis of NF is made before the patient develops toxic shock.

Necrotizing Fasciitis Throughout History

Cases of necrotizing fasciitis can be found sporadically throughout history, starting as early as the fifth century B.C. when Hippocrates, the father of medicine, made the following observations:

Many were attacked by the erysipelas [a type of skin infection] all over the body when the exciting cause was a trivial accident. . . . Flesh, sinews, and bones fell away in large quantities. . . . There were many deaths. The course of the disease was the same to whatever part of the body it spread. But the most dangerous cases . . . were when the pubes and genital organs were attacked.

Since then, there have been references to this disease among various historical and medical documents. The name and the degree of attention changes, but it's the same disease.

NF was already well documented in the medical community by the mid-1800s, according to Dr. Alfred Jay Bollet of the Yale University School of Medicine. In his book *Civil War Medicine: Unsung Battles for Life,* Dr. Bollet reports that NF—or "hospital gangrene," as it was known at that time—was the most feared and deadly wound infection of nineteenth century. Throughout the Civil War, hospital gangrene spread like wildfire among wounded soldiers, exacerbated by the lack of knowledge on the part of physicians about how infectious diseases were spread. Amputations of limbs were commonplace. Nearly half the infected soldiers—over 2,600 men—lost their lives to the disease.

According to Dr. Bollet, during the Crimean War a decade earlier (1853–1856), the rapid spread of the disease "along the French forces was described as raging 'with extraordinary virulence and fatality among the French in the hospitals on the Bosporus [an important trade route].' A French hospital ship, the *Euphrate,* enforced the extreme form of isolation, since, 'in her voyage to the Mediterranean [the crew] was obliged, from this cause alone, to throw sixty men overboard within thirty-six hours!'"

Since then, NF has been called by many other names, such as strep gangrene, phagedena (meaning "eating away"), phagedenic gangraenosa, necrotizing subcutaneous infection, and suppurative fasciitis. In 1952, the term *necrotizing fasciitis* was first published in the medical literature by a Dr. Wilson and was eventually adopted by the medical community as the most accurate term for the disease.

In the years since, while NF has remained a comparatively rare disease, it has by no means gone unnoticed in the medical literature. In fact, since 1967, over 800 articles about NF have been published in various international medical and research journals, over 70 percent of them since 1988.

Public Awareness of Necrotizing Fasciitis

It wasn't until 1989 that necrotizing fasciitis first made headline news across the United States in the wake of an article by Dr. Dennis Stevens about the disease published in *The New England Journal of Medicine*. Over 400 articles appeared across the United States including those in *Newsweek, Redbook,* and *Ladies' Home Journal.* Mainstream television programs that also covered the story, included *CBS Nightly News.* NF was also tagged in the British tabloids as the "killer bug," increasing interest and exposure throughout the world. Then clusters of invasive group A strep infections and multiple cases of NF were reported in England, Canada, and throughout the United States. In 1988, twenty cases were reported in the Rocky Mountain area. In 1992, eleven people fell victim to the disease in Gloucestershire, England. In 1994, the premier of Quebec, Lucien Bouchard, was stricken with NF, resulting in the amputation of his left leg. In 1997, two outbreaks in the United States made national headlines, causing near panic in their respective states. Texas reported over 250 cases of invasive group A strep infections resulting in forty-five deaths, many of them children. In the same year in Rochester, New York, nineteen people were stricken with invasive group A strep, with two deaths attributed to NF.

NF in the News: From Fact to Fiction

As the public's concern grew regarding necrotizing fasciitis, so did the attention from television news, tabloid magazines, and even mainstream publications. One story after another was released, each more shocking than the last and, unfortunately, most creeping ever further from fact toward fiction. One such story intimated that the flesh-eating bacteria was brought to this country by illegal aliens from other countries—an unfair and inaccurate statement indeed. However, to satisfy the human need to place blame, this speculative and unsupported statement, as well as others, found fertile ground in many communities.

Sensational news reports like "THE FLESH-EATING BACTERIA ATE MY FACE!" in far-off locations continued to astound and frighten people, young and old alike. But then victims of the disease began cropping up in our own communities—from sleepy, seaside villages in Maine, to rural towns in Kansas, to congested cities such as Los Angeles, California. Fueled by the myths and half-truths being reported in the tabloids, many terrified people avoided hospitals and yanked their children out of school for fear of their becoming infected. All at once, so it appeared, the human race was being invaded by an alien disease that devoured human flesh like a frenzy of microscopic piranhas would, while doctors stood helplessly by, powerless to stop it.

The Void of Information

At each new wave of publicity, the CDC in Atlanta, Georgia, and local health departments were swamped with frantic phone calls. The public wanted answers to countless questions—everything from "What are the symptoms of this disease?" to "Is this an epidemic?" The state and federal health departments did their best to field the thousands of phone calls, but there was no organization in existence that would offer education and support to which they could refer their frightened callers. Even the Internet, the seemingly endless universe of information, had nothing to offer.

This void of information became painfully apparent to us, the authors, as survivors of NF. When we piloted the National Necrotizing Fasciitis Foundation online at www.nnff.org in May of 1997, we were bombarded with e-mail and messages from grateful people from all over the world who finally had somewhere to turn when NF suddenly and mercilessly invaded their lives. As of this writing, more than 130,000 people have contacted us via the Web site—often thousands at a time after a national broadcast regarding the disease.

And the rumors and mistruths about NF continue to run rampant.

For example, in the early months of 2000, necrotizing fasciitis became the subject of a worldwide Internet hoax, which claimed that bananas imported from Costa Rica were infected with necrotizing fasciitis. The e-mail was quite believable for the general public, and even as of this writing, it continues to snowball. The unwitting "originator" of the e-mail—a woman who received the warning about "flesh-eating bananas" from a friend in Costa Rica and whose name, e-mail address, and business phone number were included at the bottom of the text—told us that she received over 500 e-mails and more than 300 telephone calls per day from frantic people demanding to know if the report was true.

To help dispel the public's fears, we published a disclaimer on the NNFF Web site and received over 30,000 visitors in only a couple of months. The CDC was inundated as well, and to dispel the public's fear, the Centers made the hoax headline news on their National Center for Infectious Diseases Web site. Many national media organizations also covered the hoax, including *Salon* magazine, the Associated Press, and several talk shows on National Public Radio. Unfortunately, the fruit industry was forced to address the hoax as well, as the magnitude of the public's fear unfairly threatened sales of produce.

Necrotizing Fasciitis and Popular Programs

In the late 1990s, NF began surfacing as a subject on popular television and radio programs. For example, in September of 1998, the hit television show *Guinness World Records Primetime* featured NF in a highly graphic, stomach-wrenching segment. It gave NF the dubious honor of being "the world's worst flesh-eating bacteria." Our toll-free number and Web site were bombarded after the show aired.

In March of 1998, popular Nevada-based radio call-in talk show host and author Art Bell featured the flesh-eating bacteria as the topic for discussion on his weekly show *Coast to Coast*. Though extraterrestrials, crop circles, psychic phenomena, government conspiracies, and similar otherworldly topics are most often the subjects du jour for Mr. Bell, at the time, the "outbreak" in Texas was in full swing. With 400 stations carrying the show throughout the United States, millions tuned in.

There were over 12,000 visitors to our Web site in less than twenty-four hours following that broadcast, 22,000 in only a few weeks.

Necrotizing fasciitis has been featured on the popular series *X-Files*, the popular cartoon *The Simpsons*, and the television dramas *Chicago Hope*, *The Practice*, and *L.A. Doctors*. It seems like a new and cutting-edge topic, but as you have read, despite the recent media attention, necrotizing fasciitis is not a new disease. On the contrary, NF is a very old disease, simply sporting a new nickname.

Other Types of Necrotizing Soft-Tissue Infections

NF is just one category of necrotizing soft-tissue infection (NSTI). There are other types, which are categorized based on the depth of soft-tissue involvement or the type of organism causing the infection. See Figure 1.1 for the different levels of soft tissue and their correlating NSTIs that we will discuss. The medical treatment for all categories of NSTI remains quite similar to that of NF, as we touched upon earlier, and as we will describe in great detail in Chapter 6 of this book.

Necrotizing Cellulitis

Necrotizing cellulitis is a progressing infection that affects the subcutaneous fat, sparing destruction of the deep fasciae. It is sometimes a complication of untreated or inadequately treated cellulitis, a skin infection often caused by group A streptococci and/or the bacterium *Staphylococcus aureus*. The symptoms of cellulitis and NF are often identical in the earliest stages, and distinguishing between them can be tricky for physicians.

Necrotizing Myositis

Also known as myonecrosis and gas gangrene, necrotizing myositis is a deeper necrotizing soft-tissue infection that attacks the muscle. Typically associated with a bacterium known as clostridium, this highly dangerous infection is often a complication of trauma, such as a crushing injury or surgery, particularly of the gastrointestinal or genitourinary tract. The symptoms are similar to those of NF—flulike symptoms, extreme pain, and confusion—although those of necrotizing myositis can be much more severe and rapidly spreading. An extremely foul odor is associated with this type of necrotizing soft-tissue infection, as is crepitus, a crackling sound caused by the presence of gas in the subcutaneous tissues. As is the case with NF, early diagnosis, surgical intervention, and massive doses of antibiotics are necessary to save the life of the patient.

☙

The key to shattering the contemporary myths that surround NF, is awareness and education for both our medical doctors and ourselves—a point we will make often. The fact that you're reading this book now is a significant step in that direction.

So, now that you know what necrotizing fasciitis is, as well as its history to date, let's turn to the next chapter, which will explain just how NF is contracted.

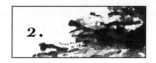

2.

How Necrotizing Fasciitis Is Contracted

EVERY moment of our lives, our bodies are engaged in a well-organized, highly effective war against millions of potentially dangerous microscopic organisms that live all around us. Most of the time, the immune system's amazing ability to fend off menacing bacteria and viruses is so great that we have no inkling that we were ever in any danger. However, sometimes our bodies are unable to protect us, and we become ill due to any number of bacterial and/or viral infections, such as the common cold, influenza, and, rarely, necrotizing fasciitis.

In this chapter we will highlight the various types of bacteria that are historically responsible for causing necrotizing fasciitis. We will also explore how the bacteria that cause NF attack once they're allowed to enter the body. Special attention will be given to group A streptococcus, a microorganism capable of causing one of the fastest and most deadly types of necrotizing infection. We will also describe just how the bacterium does its devastating damage as it causes necrotizing fasciitis.

Overview of the Bacteria That Cause NF

As mentioned in Chapter 1, several different types of bacteria can cause NF. When only one bacterium is involved, it is known as pure, or monomicrobial, necrotizing fasciitis. Group A streptococcus is the most common cause of monomicrobial NF. A case caused by two or more different kinds of bacteria is classified as a synergistic, polymicrobial, or mixed necrotizing fasciitis. Polymicrobial infections are the more common causes of NF.

Some bacteria, classified as aerobic, must have oxygen to thrive and multiply. Others, anaerobic bacteria, do not. It is possible for both anaerobic and aerobic bacteria jointly to cause necrotizing fasciitis. As we will discuss later in this book, a mixed infection of anaerobic and aerobic bacteria causes gas in the subcutaneous tissues, which is detectable by CTSCAN or MRI, while NF caused by group A strep alone does not.

The type of bacteria that causes NF frequently correlates to an underlying condition or situation. For example, *Bacteroides,* a genus of bacteria normally found in the intestines, and *Staphylococcus aureus* are common causes of NF in those who are suffering from diabetes, while group A streptococcus is often the cause of NF in young, otherwise healthy individuals or those in which no apparent trauma is discovered. Prevotella is often the cause of NF that affects the mouth and face. This correlation is significant in helping physicians as they struggle against the clock to diagnose necrotizing fasciitis properly and determine the cause in order to tailor the appropriate antibiotic therapy and other treatments.

In the following paragraphs we will highlight the most common of the various types of bacteria that have historically been identified as causes of necrotizing fasciitis.

Invasive Group A Streptococci

Streptococci are categorized according to their appearance and structure. Group A streptococci are the most pathogenic group to humans. Invasive group A streptococci are among the most predominant causes of necrotizing fasciitis. It may surprise you to learn that the group A strep bacteria are so common that one in five of us is carrying them in our noses and throats and on our skin at this very moment, often without showing any symptoms. Children carry group A strep in their throats more often than do adults. As of this writing there are over 100 variations of group A strep bacteria, called serotypes.

Infection with noninvasive group A strep bacteria is the cause of pharyngitis (infection of the pharynx, which is located at the back of the mouth), strep throat, and often impetigo. Complications from a group A strep infection can lead to rheumatic fever and post-streptococcal glomerulonephritis, a serious affliction of the kidneys that can occur ten to fourteen days after infection.

Invasive group A streptococcal bacteria, however, penetrate the body through the blood, lungs, or openings in the skin, causing severe and life-threatening illnesses such as pneumonia, meningitis, septicemia (infection of the blood), cellulitis, necrotizing fasciitis, and streptococcal toxic shock syndrome (STSS—a swiftly progressing infection that shuts down internal organs such as the liver, lungs, and kidneys). Sometimes necrotizing fasciitis can occur in conjunction with streptococcal toxic shock syndrome (NF-STSS), sharply accelerating the speed and deadliness of the infection.

Staphylococcus Aureus

Staphylococcus aureus is the most lethal of the staphylococcal bacteria. Like strep A, it can be carried on our skin or in our noses at any given time without causing symptoms. It is the culprit behind many types of infections ranging from mild to severe, including boils, carbuncles, and food poisoning. *Staphylococcus aureus* is also a major cause of wound and hospital-acquired infections, endocarditis (inflammation of the lining of the heart and its valves), and bacteremia (infection of the blood). *Staphylococcus aureus* is usually part of polymicrobial necrotizing fasciitis.

Bacteroides

Bacteroides are anaerobic bacteria, meaning they thrive without the presence of oxygen. They normally reside in the mouth, intestines, and genitals. Like *Staphylococcus aureus, Bacteroides* generally cause NF in conjunction with other types of bacteria.

Clostridium

Clostridium is a highly dangerous anaerobic genus of bacteria that feeds on decayed plant or animal tissue. Normally, it is found in the soil and some-

A Flesh-Eating . . . Fungus? The Facts about Other Conditions That Mimic NF

We receive phone calls and e-mail all the time that at first seem out-landish but, upon investigation, are loosely based in fact—like the title of this inset. Is there such a thing as a flesh-eating fungus? Well, not *exactly.* Read on for the real story.

Mucormycosis

Mucormycosis is a highly fatal infection caused by various airborne fungi of the *Mucorales* order, commonly found in bread and fruit mold. Mu-cormycosis rarely infects humans; however, when it does, those who are severely immunocompromised, such as severe burn patients and those suffering from complications from diabetes, HIV, or leukemia, are at highest risk.

Mucormycosis mimics NF in many ways, including causing rapidly spreading soft tissue necrosis and bullae. Like necrotizing fasciitis, mu-cormycosis requires early diagnosis, extensive surgical debridement, and sometimes amputation to save the life of the patient. Mucormycosis is known to affect the sinuses and soft palate and can spread very quickly to affect the brain.

Vibrio Vulnificus

Vibrio vulnificus is a bacterium that occurs naturally in estuarine waters, residing in high numbers in filter-feeding shellfish such as oysters, clams, and mussels. According to Dr. James Oliver, professor of biology at the University of North Carolina at Charlotte and a leading expert on the bac-terium, the organism causes infection in people through ingestion, such as eating raw oysters, or through a wound, such as cutting or puncturing the hand while shucking oysters, peeling shrimp, or cleaning fish. Most often, people with underlying illnesses—especially liver or blood dis-eases—are at highest risk for falling ill due to this bacterium following in-gestion. In contrast, people who develop wound infections from this organism typically do not have underlying disease. The wound infections in people who do have liver or blood disorders typically progress rapidly and become systemic, often resulting in amputation. Death occurs in 25 percent of wound cases. In a recent study of soft-tissue infections in Florida, the great majority (82 percent) of those that resulted in death was caused by *Vibrio vulnificus.* Although all persons are susceptible, most wound infections occur in men aged forty-five or older. *Vibrio vulnificus* is the cause of 95 percent of all seafood-related deaths in the United States.

Vibrio vulnificus infections of the skin often develop into necrotizing soft-tissue infections, causing such symptoms as inflammation, fever, and extensive tissue destruction at the location of the inciting wound. Prompt diagnosis, powerful antibiotics, and surgical management are necessary to save the life of the patient.

Brown Recluse Spider Bite

The bite of the brown recluse spider, also known as the fiddleback or *Loxosceles reclusa,* can also cause localized skin and soft tissue necrosis and is sometimes confused with necrotizing fasciitis. In the hours after a bite, a lesion appears resembling a bull's-eye—it has a blue circle with red interior. This lesion is often accompanied by rash, lethargy, fever, and chills. The spider's venom can also cause the victim's skin and subcutaneous tissue to necrose, forming a deep, painful ulceration surrounded by reddened, inflamed tissue. Treatment includes antibiotics and wound care; however, the bite is rarely fatal.

The brown recluse spider is fond of warm, dry climates; however, it can be found throughout the United States.

times in the intestines of humans and animals. It causes diseases like botulism, a severe type of food poisoning, and tetanus, a disease that attacks the nervous system. *Clostridium perfringens, Clostridium histolylicum,* and *Clostridium septicum* are not as common causes of NF as is group A strep, but they are causes of gas gangrene, a rapidly progressing fatal necrotizing infection that may occur following penetrating trauma or a crushing injury in patients with low white blood counts or cancer of the colon.

Pseudomonads

Pseudomonads bacteria are responsible for a wide range of infections from mild to severe, including skin infections and pneumonia and other respiratory infections, depending on the underlying health of the host. The genus *Pseudomonas* is often blamed for NF in patients with severely compromised immune systems.

Prevotella

Prevotella is a genus of anaerobic bacteria that can exist throughout the body without causing symptoms. *Prevotella* is typically discovered to be a cause of NF cases in the mouth, jaw, neck, and face, usually in association with other bacteria.

How NF Bacteria Are Contracted

Believe it or not, the process by which a person contracts NF is not simple. As mentioned earlier, our bodies have several barriers against infection, including our skin and our immune systems. In order for a person to contract necrotizing fasciitis, two things must happen. First, invasive bacteria must have an opportunity to enter the body. This often happens through a break or weakening in the skin, such as a cut, bruise, or postsurgical incision, although spontaneous infections, in which no inciting injury can be found, are also possible. A person must then be directly exposed to the microorganisms that cause NF—either with the bacteria residing on their own bodies or through direct contact with a person carrying the bacteria. However, keep in mind that this does not necessarily mean that the person will then develop necrotizing fasciitis. In fact, more often than not, he or she does not. Once the bacteria gain entry into the body, damage occurs quite swiftly. As they rapidly reproduce, the bacteria release toxins and enzymes into the surrounding tissues. These toxins and enzymes incite the body's inflammatory response, causing pain, swelling, and fever.

Group A Streptococcus

As you learned earlier in this chapter, group A strep causes strep throat and other non–life-threatening illnesses, in addition to necrotizing fasciitis. However, it is possible for a person carrying group A strep (with or without symptoms) to pass the infection along to another human being, at which point, due to a break in the skin, the infection becomes invasive. Necrotizing fasciitis can then develop. Read the following story as told by "Sally."

> I remember that my children and I were very sick with strep throat. My two-year-old was inconsolable, and so his father, "Mark," was holding him, trying to rock him to sleep. Mark was the only one in the household who was not battling a fever and sore throat. The next day, however, Mark felt horrible—sick to his stomach and he had extreme pain in his arm and shoulder. The only injury he had was a cut on his finger—nothing unusual in his job as a chef. He grew steadily worse, and finally he agreed to let us bring him to the emergency room. We spent hours waiting to see a doctor. Suddenly, while he was being examined, Mark's system completely shut down. A day and half later, Mark was dead from toxic shock caused by necrotizing fasciitis.

Group A strep is transferred from person to person on exhaled respiratory droplets. Remember growing up when your mother continually told you to cover your mouth when you coughed or to cover your nose when you sneezed? Not only is it polite, but it can help prevent the dangerous spread of germs. Remember that one in five of us carries strep A at any given time. When we sneeze, the bacteria are propelled into the air on droplets. In fact, sneezing is a defense mechanism designed to expel germs from the body—at a rate of as many as 5,000 droplets at a time, traveling as far as 3.7 meters (over twelve feet)! The bacteria are then easily picked up by the next person walking in the path of the droplets or are transferred via direct contact, like a handshake. The same scenario is true with coughing and children wiping noses with their hands. If a person breathes in the bacteria, he or she may become ill with strep throat. If he or she has a cut or scratch and the bacteria gain entry, a necrotizing infection can occur.

However, unlike airborne diseases, the respiratory droplets contaminated with group A strep do not remain suspended in the air. Contrary to some reports, group A strep infection is not an airborne germ but a disease contracted by contact with respiratory droplets of an infected individual. The distinction between the two merits an explanation of airborne infectious diseases.

An airborne infectious disease is one in which minute droplets containing the infectious microorganisms remain suspended in the air for an extended time. It may also be carried on microscopic dust particles, which float freely through the air to be inhaled by or deposited on an unwitting human being whether they are near the infected individual or not. Examples of microorganisms spread by airborne transmission are tuberculosis and varicella (chickenpox.)

Group A strep can be passed along on inanimate objects, but only in circumstances where perhaps someone sneezes, transfers the bacteria to their hand, and then transfers the bacteria to a door handle. Should a person with an open wound touch that door handle, he or she could be infected shortly thereafter.

It's important to realize the difference between group A strep bacteria infections and necrotizing fasciitis. When the media speaks of group A strep outbreaks, this does not necessarily mean that it is an outbreak of the "flesh-eating bacteria." It means that there has been a concentration of cases in a geographical area of group A strep infections. Out of these cases, none or only a small percentage are actually necrotizing fasciitis.

NF caused by group A strep is a particularly virulent, rapidly progressing infection often occurring in association with streptococcal toxic shock syndrome. If it weren't so deadly, the speed and ferocity of necrotizing fasciitis caused by group A strep would be awesome to behold. The disease can visibly spread up a victim's leg or arm in hours, destroying all of the tissue in its path. What makes group A strep in particular such a virulent infection? How does it travel so quickly? And why doesn't the immune system do more to contain the infection? We'll try to answer these questions and more in the following paragraphs.

Group A strep, like many bacteria that cause disease, produce substances that help protect them from the human immune defenses and facilitate their entry into deeper tissues. Infection by group A strep is a battle between the organism and the body's natural defenses. One of the major proteins on the surface of the bacteria is called the M protein. This is one of the substances that allow the organism to survive in the hostile human environment. The M protein can serve as an anchor to attach the bacteria to the cells of the throat or skin. When the infection begins, the M protein also helps disguise the bacteria from the immune cells that would otherwise ingest and kill it. M proteins accomplish this in part by binding with normal human serum proteins, which mask the otherwise foreign bacterial surface. In other words, once the organism invades the body, it takes on a surface coat that looks like human proteins instead of bacterial substances. Group A strep also make several proteins that specifically bind to or digest some components of the immune system. As a result of all of these strep products, the bacteria can enter the host and will not immediately be killed by the host's defense systems.

Group A strep also produce a number of toxins that facilitate entry of the bacteria into tissues and cause an inflammatory response. The symptoms of infection are due in large part to the inflammatory response to the organism as well as the presence of the organism itself. Group A strep also produces certain enzymes that cause tissue damage as well as inhibit the clotting system, enabling the bacteria to move more freely through tissues.

Students of the bacterium marvel at its ability to maintain, in most cases, the delicate balance between causing infection and permitting its host to survive. For if the infection were life threatening at all times, the bacterium would soon find that it had no hosts remaining. For this reason some think that the life-threatening cases of infection are accidents along the path of the evolutionary relationship of bacteria and host. After all, there is no real long-term advantage for the group A strep bacterium that kills its host.

Staphylococcus Aureus

While group A strep is contracted by droplet transmission, *Staphylococcus aureus* is contracted by direct contact with infected persons or objects. If a health-care worker is carrying *Staphylococcus aureus* and handles a patient, the bacteria are easily transferred to that patient. *Staphylococcus aureus* can also be transferred to inanimate objects such as gloves, needles, and blood pressure monitoring equipment, where it can be picked up by patients or health-care workers. It is the most prevalent nosocomial and postoperative infection.

Outside the hospital, *Staphylococcus aureus* is responsible for a large percentage of wound infections. These infections may be caused by *Staphylococcus aureus* already existing on the skin or being allowed to enter the wound through a contaminated object. Dishes, silverware, fabrics, toys, and countertops can become contaminated with *Staphylococcus aureus,* aiding in its transmission to human beings.

Due to the fact that *Staphylococcus aureus* resides in and around the perineum (the area in and around the anus and genitalia), it can cause an invasive gangrenous infection of the genitalia (in conjunction with anaerobic bacteria) known as Fournier's gangrene. This horrifying infection often begins as a painful boil in the area of the perineum but progresses to engulf the entire pubic area of the patient, causing inflammation, swelling, fever, extreme pain, and gangrene. Aggressive debridement and removal of sexual organs is not uncommon. *Staphylococcus aureus* can also be associated with a less aggressive form of NF. As mentioned previously, it is known to cause NF in conjunction with other types of bacteria.

&

If you're a survivor of necrotizing fasciitis or know the pain of watching a loved one struggle to survive NF, it may be very difficult to believe that this devastating disease has such a mundane origin. Nevertheless, as we've explained in this chapter, the bacteria that cause NF are very much a part of our everyday lives. They can invade the body by entering an opening in the skin as trivial as a paper cut. They can strike anyone, at any time, whether considered at risk or not.

However, if you are just learning the facts about this disease, don't use this information to create a life filled with fear. Every cough and sneeze in a crowded airplane, elevator, or restaurant must not create instant panic in you about catching the "killer bug." And while it is certainly understandable for our readers who have been affected by NF to be more cautious in their daily lives, it is important to remember that NF is very rare, and unlikely to strike again.

In the next chapter we'll explain the different opportunities for NF to enter the body, and who is at higher risk of contracting the disease.

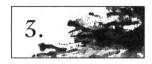

Opportunities for Infection and Higher-Risk Groups

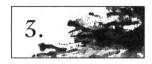

As YOU should know by now, necrotizing fasciitis does not discriminate in selecting its victims. None of us is immune from the possibility of contracting the disease, whether we are healthy or not. However, there are certain higher-risk conditions and situations that can be ideal opportunities for a necrotizing soft-tissue infection. In this chapter we will identify these higher-risk situations and briefly explain the reasons for the increased danger.

In about half of all NF cases, the bacteria enter the body through a weakness in the skin. The remaining 50 percent of NF cases are defined as spontaneous—no entry point can be identified.

Recent Wounds

On the job, in the home, on the playground, and in the yard, few things are more common than the daily minor bumps, bruises, cuts, and scratches. We often give the injury a passing thought and then forget all about it. But the frightening truth is that what seem like insignificant injuries are the leading points of origin of the organisms that cause necrotizing fasciitis, particularly rapidly spreading group A strep bacteria, which attack otherwise healthy, vibrant people.

"Timothy" is a lovable, curious seventeen-month-old boy. One day while exploring, he pulled on a heavy kitchen chair and it caught his foot, leaving a tiny scratch on his left little toe. Within the hour, the toddler's foot was swelling. Within twenty-four hours, Timothy was fighting a fever of 103 degrees and his foot was turning black with pus oozing from the scratch on his little toe. His worried mom, "Gail," took him to the emergency room, thinking that her son's foot was broken. The X-rays were normal. However, the boy's bloodwork revealed a very high white blood cell count of 20,000. Timothy was admitted and immediately given intravenous antibiotics. During his six-day hospital stay, he underwent six operations to remove infected tissue. He was finally released, although he still needed intravenous antibiotics and skilled nursing visits daily to change wound dressings.

"I am just amazed at how many people this is affecting," Gail told us. "I had seen this [necrotizing fasciitis] on either *60 Minutes* or *Dateline,* but thought that it could never happen around here. Boy, was I wrong! I am a nervous wreck now that my family will get a cut or scratch and get the bacteria, since we have no idea where it came from in the first place."

The minor injuries that can precede NF are limited only by the imagination. The following is a list of some actual injuries that have resulted in severe, if not fatal, bouts with necrotizing fasciitis:

- A banged foot on the bed during the night
- A boil on the inner thigh
- A bruise on the arm caused by a friendly punch from a friend
- A leg bumped on a golf bag
- A carpet burn
- A cat bite on the toe
- A caught finger in a zipper while closing a suitcase
- A cut finger on electrical wire
- A cut finger on a staple
- An abrasion on elbow or leg after slipping on ice

- An ingrown hair in the groin area
- A needle prick from a blood test
- A puncture in the palm from a poultry bone while preparing dinner
- Scratched insect bites
- A small rash on the leg
- A spider bite on the forearm
- A sprained ankle

NF caused by recent wounds tends to be the most difficult for physicians to diagnose. Often the patient has no reason to believe that a tiny paper cut or an ingrown hair could be in any way related to their symptoms, which may include severe limb pain and swelling, high fever, vomiting, diarrhea, and dehydration. Consequently, when the patient seeks medical attention for his or her symptoms, he or she does not report the injury. This contributes to the missed and/or delayed diagnosis of NF.

Conversely, sometimes the patient points out the injury to the physician, but the doctor doesn't make the connection between the minor injury and the symptoms until the patient's condition becomes critical and the damage to the body becomes irreparable. Unfortunately, this happens often. In Chapter 5, you will read more about the widespread problem of missed and/or delayed diagnosis of NF.

Recent Surgical Procedures

If you've ever had surgery, chances are that you remember signing a consent form that indicated that postoperative infection, among other things, was within the realm of possibility after the operation. All surgical procedures, from elective to emergency, carry an inherent risk of infection for several reasons. Any surgical procedure can serve as an entry point for NF bacteria. The most common procedures, however, include abdominal surgery, cesarean section for delivery of a baby, vaginal childbirth, and oral surgery.

Despite stringent measures to ensure sterile conditions, bacteria can never be fully eradicated from the operating room. Surgical wounds can become infected with bacteria residing on the patient's own skin.

Surgical instruments such as scalpels and clamps may be contaminated, and personnel in the operating room may be carrying invasive bacteria. To add to the problem, the surgical patient may be suffering from an underlying illness that renders the immune system ineffective in fighting off invasive bacteria. Following is the story of how "Carol" contracted NF after her surgery.

Carol underwent minor surgery, which was performed on both of her breasts. Not long after she was discharged from the hospital, she began to develop unusual redness around her wounds, a fever of about 101°F, and lower back pains. She called her doctor, who was out of town, and was told by her doctor's associate that she probably had a virus. The doctor told her to monitor her symptoms and to call back if they worsened. As the day progressed, her temperature continued to rise, and she began to feel nauseous. The doctor tried changing Carol's pain medication, thinking that her nausea was a reaction to the drugs, but by the next day her temperature had soared to 103.2°F. In addition, her breasts were swollen, increasingly reddening, and blistering; she was experiencing flulike symptoms; and she was vomiting severely. Clearly quite ill, she called the doctor's office yet again. The doctor told her to call the office on Monday (this was Saturday), when her primary physician who was familiar with her case would have returned. However, by Monday, Carol was quite concerned, so rather than calling the doctor, she went to the doctor's office first thing Monday morning.

When the doctors saw the condition of her breasts, they were, of course, immediately concerned, and her physician promptly admitted her to the hospital for exploratory surgery in order to determine the cause of her symptoms. When she awakened following surgery, she learned that both of her breasts had been removed because so much of her breast tissue was necrotic. After speaking with her treating infectious disease specialist, she learned that she had contracted a somewhat rare postoperative infection, necrotizing fasciitis, caused by group A strep bacteria—the "flesh-eating bacteria."

Carol has since undergone more than twenty reconstructive surgical procedures because breast reconstruction was so difficult due to the loss of so much tissue and muscle. In addition to her first complicating strep infection, she had subsequently suffered from several staph infections in her wounds due to insufficient blood flow to the area. More than two years later, she is still trying to recover from the first relatively minor surgery.

Prior to surgery, doctors will often order preventive antibiotic regimens (called prophylaxis) to help prevent infection. This regimen may continue after the surgery as well. Yet, in spite of prophylactic antibiotics, the risk of infection remains with the patient throughout the entire recovery period, whether they are hospitalized or recuperating at home.

Hospital-Acquired Infections

An infection acquired in the hospital is known as a nosocomial infection. Despite sterile procedures, hospitals are hotbeds for infections, and they appear to be getting worse. In fact, the Centers for Disease Control's (CDC's) National Nosocomial Infections Surveillance (NNIS) system reports that nosocomial infections in the United States have increased 36 percent in the past twenty years.

According to reports, each year over two million people contract hospital-acquired infections, resulting in over 88,000 deaths—one death every six minutes. Patients in intensive care units (ICUs), as well as the obstetrical/gynecological sections, are much more likely to fall victim to nosocomial infections. *Staphylococcus aureus* and group A strep, leading causes of NF, are common causes of nosocomial infections.

With all the recent advancements in technology, medicine, and education, why on earth would hospital infections be on the increase? According to "Nosocomial Infection Update," an article written by Dr. Robert Weinstein and published in the fall of 1998 in the CDC's publication *Emerging Infectious Diseases,* there are three cooperative forces contributing to the problem: antibiotic-resistant microbes, lax infection-control procedures, and the increasing number of outpatient procedures.

Antibiotic-Resistant Microbes

Before doctors realized the problem with antibiotic-resistant microbes, antibiotics were prescribed in ever-increasing numbers to patients for a variety of afflictions—often unnecessarily. In a textbook example of Darwin's theory of "survival of the fittest," microorganisms that were once successfully treated with antibiotics have intelligently mutated so that they are now capable of shrugging off the effects of these "wonder drugs."

To cite an example, one particularly crafty form of *Staphylococcus aureus* that is outwitting even our highest-powered weapon—an antibiotic called vancomycin—has evolved. This particular bug, which is called vancomycin-resistant *Staphylococcus aureus* (VRSA), is currently undergoing extensive study by researchers in an effort to find a way to fight back.

Lax Infection Control Procedures

A good percentage of nosocomial infections could be thwarted by the enforcement of fundamental infection control procedures, such as washing hands between patient contacts. "Wait a minute now," you may be thinking, "don't doctors and nurses wash their hands after touching a sick patient?" Unfortunately, not always. The CDC and other infectious diseases committees have recognized this problem in recent years and have issued a flurry of directives to encourage hand-washing and other infection-control procedures among health-care workers. Often in the ICU, where nosocomial infections are most prevalent, a conflict often exists between saving a patient's life and taking the time to change gloves or wash hands. To illustrate this point, imagine a child recovering from open-heart surgery in the pediatric ICU. All of a sudden, in an already chaotic ward, monitors scream and alarms blare as the child goes into cardiac arrest. Doctors and nurses in the midst of working with another critical-care patient spring into action to save the child's life. While in nonemergency times washing hands and changing gloves are an ingrained reflex, in a situation that requires split-second response, the duty and desire to save the child's life take precedent in the minds of the physicians and nurses.

More Outpatient Procedures

"The shift of surgical care to outpatient centers leaves the sickest patients in hospitals, which are becoming more like large ICUs," explains Dr.

Weinstein. The sicker the patient, the lower the immune system defenses are, and thus the more susceptible to infection the person is. When most of the patients in the hospitals are serious candidates for infection to begin with, the statistical numbers for hospital-acquired infections rise.

Some may argue after reading about nosocomial infections that patients are far better off being allowed to recover in the comfort of their own homes after surgery. This is a good point. Resistant and invasive bacteria can be avoided, as can the psychological trauma of being separated from loved ones. However, readmission of same-day surgery patients due to complications and infections is common. Patients and family members in charge of wound care at home take on an enormous responsibility. They must be fully educated regarding the signs of infection, as well as in effectively communicating subjective symptoms to physicians over the telephone. We'll discuss this important topic in detail in later chapters.

Self-Acquired NF

We contract NF from direct contact with infected individuals, but is it possible to infect ourselves? The answer is yes. Since we carry group A strep, *Staphylococcus aureus,* and many other types of bacteria on and in our bodies at any given time, it is not hard to imagine how we could infect ourselves.

Consider the experience of Donna Batdorff. Her nearly fatal bout with NF began while on a ski trip in Colorado. First, she thought she had the flu. The next day, she noticed a tiny cut on her finger. Throughout the next few days her symptoms rapidly progressed from annoying muscle pain to severe nausea and diarrhea, extreme weakness. She made it back to Michigan, where she was hospitalized, and she collapsed into a coma.

According to Dr. Ben Schwartz, an epidemiologist of the Centers for Disease Control, "Donna could have come in contact with someone who had it, or had it herself in her throat."

Spontaneous Necrotizing Fasciitis Infections

Approximately 50 percent of NF cases are defined as *spontaneous,* in which no entry point can be identified. Spontaneous NF is often associated with a lightning-fast, highly fatal necrotizing infection coupled with streptococcal toxic shock syndrome, a topic we'll cover later in the chapter. The following story of Ray is an example of how swiftly spontaneous necrotizing fasciitis can progress.

On Wednesday evening my husband, Ray, said he really wasn't hungry for the dinner I had prepared, which wasn't like him. I asked if he was feeling all right. "Yes," he replied, "I'm just not hungry." That night I took his temperature. It was a bit elevated, but I thought he was just getting a bug. The next evening he had a slight fever, and his right hand hurt him a little. I gave him aspirin and we went to bed. When I woke at 6:15 Friday morning, I noticed Ray wasn't in bed. I found him sitting on the couch in the living room. "I just couldn't sleep," he explained. "My hand hurts so much." The hand was still swollen and had turned bright red. He grew weak very quickly. I decided to take him to the hospital. By the time we reached it, Ray couldn't even get out of the car. The security guard helped us get him into a wheelchair and into the emergency unit.

Paperwork followed, along with questions and more questions. Could a spider have bitten Ray? Had he injured his hand in his workshop or in the yard? Did something happen to him while we were in vacation in Florida? All the answers were negative. He didn't go outside or into a workshop because of the arthritis, and we had been home from Florida almost three weeks.

By now Ray was writhing with pain. In addition, the nurse had discovered a very strange purple spot under his right arm. It was about two inches by three inches in size, had definite lines around it like the boundaries of a country, and was dark purple in the center. This was like nothing I had ever seen before. Tests, including ultrasound, were necessary in order to determine whether there were blood clots present. I returned to the emergency room and waited.

When Ray returned, I couldn't believe my eyes! His hand had turned into a round ball and was almost black! Huge brown blisters covered his hand and were oozing! Also, the spot under his arm had doubled in size, was swollen, and had blisters that were oozing. I became dizzy. The exact chain of events that followed is difficult to remember, but it seems the next thing I knew, Ray was headed for the operating room. I was told he had some terrible infection.

As they wheeled Ray into the operating room, his surgeon stopped me. "I'm sorry to tell you, I don't know if we can save his hand, and I don't know if we can save his life," he told me. I couldn't believe this was really happening. Last night Ray was only getting a bug, and now he may be dying?

Ray's right arm had to be amputated about four inches below the elbow, and a large section of skin and flesh was removed from the right side of his chest and under the arm. Ray was put on a ventilator and given large doses of antibiotics. I counted twelve bags of fluids hanging around his bed, dripping into his body. All of the monitors overwhelmed me. For the next ten days I lived at the hospital. Ray had necrotizing fasciitis, or the flesh-eating bacteria—something I had never heard of. Ray's kidneys had shut down but began functioning again. His heart rate shot up dramatically, and his blood pressure went way down. There were two more surgeries and debridements [surgical removal of dead flesh], and many complications during his recovery. Ray was in an induced coma for almost four weeks. After thirty-nine days in the hospital and fifteen more at a rehab center, I brought him home.

—Evelyn Holst

The disease moves with extraordinary speed, as in Ray's experience, swiftly destroying subcutaneous tissue and causing major organs of the body, such as the kidneys, liver, and lungs, to shut down. This is called streptococcal toxic shock syndrome (STSS). Spontaneous NF in conjunction with STSS (NF/STSS) is a highly fatal form of necrotizing fasciitis. The rapid advancement of symptoms from initial signs such as fever, pain, and swelling to massive tissue death and organ failure can happen overnight, leaving precious little time for doctors to diagnose and treat the disease in time to save the patient.

Underlying Conditions

In a study published in 1995 in the *Annals of Surgery,* a leading medical journal, researchers reviewed the medical records of sixty-five patients who had contracted NF, looking for underlying conditions that may have made the patients more susceptible to the disease. It was discovered that of these sixty-five people, all of them had at least one underlying condition, and 75 percent have had as many as five. Table 3.1 highlights their findings.

TABLE 3.1. PERCENTAGE OF NF PATIENTS WITH AN UNDERLYING ILLNESS IN ONE STUDY		
Underlying Condition	**Number of NF Patients with Condition**	**Percentage of Patients with Condition**
Obesity	30	46%
Diabetes mellitus	29	45%
Hypoalbuminemia (low protein, malnutrition)	26	40%
Peripheral vascular disease	17	26%
Alcoholism	8	12%
Immunosuppression	7	11%
Drug abuse	5	15%

Source: McHenry, Christopher R., M.D., et al., "Determinants of Mortality for NSTI," *Annals of Surgery,* Vol. 221, No. 5, May 1995.

While the higher-risk groups for contracting NF that we will discuss in the following paragraphs are worlds apart from each other and encompass a broad range of people (such as those suffering from alcoholism and children with chickenpox), you will begin to see several contributory factors in common. For example, in almost all of the groups, immunodeficiency is a key factor, as is malnutrition.

Alcoholics

Alcoholism is a disease that affects over 14 million people in the United States alone. According to an article in *Scientific American,* 25 to 40 percent of Americans in general hospital beds are being treated for complications of alcoholism. Alcohol is highly toxic to the system and can cause a myriad of very serious health problems due to the widespread damage it causes to cells and to the immune system. And because of damage to the liver, the organ responsible for producing digestive enzymes, the body cannot properly absorb vital nutrients, fats, and proteins, resulting in malnutrition. Adding to these already severe problems, excessive use of alcohol can cause diabetes, a higher-risk group in and of itself. The combination of a lowered immune system, malnutrition, and the development of diabetes makes individuals suffering from alcoholism more susceptible to contracting necrotizing fasciitis.

Drug Abusers

Drug abuse is a never-ending problem in the United States, affecting every corner of society—family, work, health, crime, and education. Those who abuse drugs are also at higher risk for NF because of the long-term damage that drugs have on the body. All drugs have some degree of negative effect on the immune system. In fact, habitual marijuana users can diminish their ability to defend themselves from invasive illnesses and infections by as much as 40 percent.

Intravenous drug users invite other problems that contribute to the risk of contracting necrotizing fasciitis. Chronic users of intravenous needles may develop collapsed veins, abscesses or ulcerations on the skin, and cellulitis—all perfect opportunities for developing NF. Like other infectious diseases, drug users who share needles can pass invasive bacteria to each other as well.

Drugs rob the body of essential nutrients, as well as of the ability to properly manufacture and distribute these nutrients to cells. This results in malnutrition, which forces the body into a vulnerable position when fighting illnesses.

Children with Chickenpox

Chickenpox, or varicella, is an infectious disease that most of us endured as a rite of passage during childhood. Nevertheless, chickenpox, complicated by infections such as cellulitis, necrotizing fasciitis, and toxic shock syndrome, results in approximately one hundred deaths per year in the United States, a figure that appears to be rising. In fact, complications due to chickenpox are the leading cause of death due to a disease preventable by a vaccine in children. From late 1993 to 1995, nineteen children were hospitalized at Children's Hospital and Medical Center in Seattle, Washington, due to post-varicella NF. In Texas in March of 1998, twelve cases of invasive group A strep associated with chickenpox were reported. A recent study concluded that children with chickenpox were 39 percent more likely to develop NF.

The open, oozing blisters on the skin of children suffering from chickenpox offer plenty of opportunities for invasive bacteria to gain entry into the body. Because children scratch the itchy lesions, the condition worsens. Contributing to the problem, the child's immune system is weakened due to its fight against the varicella virus. Invasive infections occur typically within two weeks of the initial onset of the disease.

There have been recent reports linking NF to the use of aspirin, ibuprofen, and other over-the-counter and prescription drugs known as nonsteroidal antiinflammatory drugs (NSAIDs) in children with chickenpox. Some physicians believe that giving children NSAIDs to treat pain and discomfort during a bout with the varicella virus exacerbates the onset of invasive bacterial infections such as necrotizing fasciitis by masking symptoms and by hampering the body's immunological response to invasive bacteria. Other physicians argue that the use of NSAIDs and the onset of invasive infections is simply coincidental. Until a correlation is established or disproved, some physicians advise erring on the side of caution by considering alternative medications (such as Tylenol) for children with chickenpox. It is worthwhile to note that the risk of necrotizing fasciitis complicating chickenpox can be avoided altogether by inoculating children with the varicella vaccine. In fact, the Centers for Disease Control has issued new federal guidelines asking each state to make the varicella vaccine mandatory for children prior to entering day care or elementary school.

> "James," a thirteen-month-old boy, came down with chicken-pox. While treating their son's lesions, James's parents noticed a large red spot on his left shoulder. Alarmed, they took him to the local hospital, where he was given Motrin for pain and was sent home. The next day the baby's arm began to worsen, with redness and swelling, so his concerned parents took him back to the hospital, where he was admitted and given intravenous antibiotics.
>
> Unfortunately, despite the fact that *in the very next bed* a little girl with chickenpox exhibiting identical symptoms had nearly lost her leg due to invasive bacteria, James's doctors chose to wait twelve hours before taking the infant into surgery. At that point the baby's left arm was rock-solid from the triceps down—a sign of dead tissue. Although, James survived, it was necessary to amputate his arm in order to contain the infection.

Those with Severe Chronic Conditions

This higher-risk group encompasses those suffering from any number of long-term severe illnesses. The predisposing factors to the increased risk of developing NF, however, remain similar: immuno-deficiency, malnutrition, exposure to infectious bacteria due to hospitalization, and sometimes impeded blood flow to tissues. Severe chronic conditions include AIDS, cancer, coronary disease, chronic renal failure, and cirrhosis of the liver, among others.

Those Undergoing Immunosuppressive Therapies

Chemotherapy, or the use of drugs to treat cancer, severely depletes the body's ability to produce white blood cells, making the patient susceptible to infections. It is especially important for patients undergoing chemotherapy to be vigilant in watching for signs of infection.

Immunosuppression is the intentional weakening of an individual's innate immune response. It is necessary for the treatment of many autoimmune conditions—conditions in which a person's immune system mistakes its own body as a foreign invader—among others, and is achieved through the use of drugs or radiation. For example, prior to organ transplant surgery, patients are treated with immunosuppressive drugs to prepare the body for the procedure. Without such treatment the immune system may react against the new tissue as it would to any intruder into the body, thus rejecting the organ.

Deliberately weakening the immune system for medical treatment can be highly valuable when necessary; however, it is clearly a threat to the patient's ability to defend him- or herself from infection. And, considering what we now know about the risk of nosocomial infections, patients recovering from invasive procedures that required immunosuppression are understandably at much higher risk of contracting NF than healthy people.

Diabetics

Diabetes is a chronic disorder in which the body's production and utilization of insulin, an essential hormone that converts sugar, starches, and other food into the energy our bodies need to function, is faulty. While researchers are at a loss as to the cause of the disease, several factors are known to contribute to the problem, including heredity, obesity, and lack of exercise.

According to the American Diabetes Association, there are 15.7 million people in the United States with diabetes. While an estimated 10.3 million have been diagnosed, unfortunately, 5.4 million people are not aware that they even have the disease. Each day, approximately 2,200 people are diagnosed with diabetes. It is the seventh leading cause of death in the United States.

People living with diabetes suffer from various complications that can become life threatening and make them vulnerable to necrotizing fasciitis. One such complication is peripheral vascular disease. Because of a thickening in the lining of blood vessels due to a buildup of sugar-based substances, blood flow is restricted to certain areas of the body. Heart disease, stroke, and kidney failure can result. Peripheral vascular disease also obstructs nourishment and disease-fighting cells from reaching the surface barriers of the body, especially the extremities. Ulcers, infection, and gangrene are common, which can often lead to necrotizing fasciitis. Peripheral neuropathy is permanent damage to the nerves of the lower extremities causing the inability to feel pressure, temperature, and pain. Because of this lack of sensation, diabetics can injure their feet and not even know it, often resulting in ulcers and infection, which can pave the way for necrotizing fasciitis. For this reason, diabetics are encouraged to meticulously care for their feet by checks for injuries daily and to avoid walking barefoot at any time.

These grave complications put individuals suffering from diabetes in jeopardy of contracting NF. Cuts, scratches, and ulcerations on the skin that go unnoticed are golden opportunities for invasive bacteria to enter the body. Once the bacteria get in, the body is unable to put up a fight due to a weakened immune system and the lack of blood flow to the tissues. And because of lack of pain sensation, the recognition of symptoms is often delayed, resulting in a lesser chance of timely diagnosis and aggressive treatment.

The Elderly

The elderly population is at greater risk of contracting necrotizing fasciitis for several reasons. As we age, our body's ability to defend itself becomes increasingly less effective, making the elderly more susceptible to contracting illnesses that in younger years would have been routinely and successfully fought off. Adding to the problem, the elderly are often hospitalized or in nursing homes or long-term care facilities with other sick individuals, where the exposure to infectious diseases is high. Furthermore, because a large percentage of elderly people live with chronic underlying conditions, such as heart disease, peripheral vascular disease, and diabetes, they are at increased risk of contracting invasive infections. Malnutrition is also an unfortunate reality among the elderly. In a recent survey of 750 physicians, nurses, and administrators of health-care institutions, it was reported that 25 percent of elderly patients are malnourished. One-half of all elderly hospital patients and 40 percent of nursing home residents are believed to suffer from malnutrition.

The Obese

Obesity is the most common chronic disorder in the United States with over one-third of the American population being overweight. Women, African-Americans, and Hispanics are more likely to be obese than others. There are many health problems attributable to obesity, including hypertension, coronary disease, non-insulin-dependent diabetes mellitus, gallbladder disease, and certain types of cancer, such as prostate cancer. One very important reason for the increased risk of NF in obese individuals is that adipose tissue, or fat, does not have a good blood supply, which in turn diminishes the body's natural disease-fighting abilities. Even a tiny injury, such as a boil or cut, is less easily defended by the immune system, leading to a greater potential of contracting NF.

Those with Peripheral Vascular Disease

In the United States over one million people suffer from peripheral vascular disease. Peripheral vascular diseases are afflictions of the blood vessels, especially in the extremities, such as arteriosclerosis—a disease that causes hardening of the arteries due to a buildup of deposits. It also includes Raynaud's disease, a circulatory disorder that makes hands and feet abnormally sensitive to cold temperatures. This disease, which is more common in women, causes the tiny blood vessels in the extremities to constrict, starving the hands and feet of oxygenated blood. Another peripheral vascular disease is thromboangiitis obliterans, also called also Buerger's disease, caused by stationary blood clots attached to the walls of small arteries and veins of the extremities.

People living with peripheral vascular disease are in greater danger of contracting invasive bacteria than healthy individuals due to the restricted flow of blood to the extremities, limiting the body's ability to fight infection.

Women Giving Birth

The process of giving birth carries inherent risks of complications to both the child and the mother, with infection being high on the list. As explained earlier, obstetrical/gynecological patients are at high risk for nosocomial infections in general. While necrotizing fasciitis in women giving birth is uncommon, it is a well-established and highly fatal occurrence that deserves special attention.

Vaginal delivery commonly causes tears in the mother's vagina, extending into the perineum. Otherwise, in order to protect the perineum from trauma and to ease the birth of the baby, physicians may perform a common surgical procedure known as an episiotomy, in which an incision is made through the skin, connective tissue, and muscle from the vagina to the rectum. Due to the proliferation of bacteria in this area of the body, in both cases, a high possibility of infection exists.

In recent years the practice of episiotomy during an otherwise normal vaginal delivery has come under repeated fire from the medical community. In fact, an article in the *American Journal of Obstetrics and Gynecology* (1996) recommends that the use of episiotomy be abandoned as the scientific evidence fails to justify its continued practice. This opinion is echoed by that of the World Health Organization, a vast network of member states of the United Nations dedicated to the worldwide prevention of disease. These recommendations strongly suggest that, in time, episiotomy could become a thing of the past. But the wheels of medical debate, mainstream acceptance, and change turn slowly, and until the final vote is in, the increased risk of infection—including necrotizing fasciitis—remains for women undergoing this procedure during childbirth.

A cesarean section (or C-section) is surgical delivery of a baby through an incision made through the abdomen and uterus. It is performed when a vaginal birth is not in the best interest of the child or mother. It requires an incision across the abdomen just above the pubic area. About 20 percent of all births in the United States are done through C-section. Like all surgical procedures, the C-section incision serves as an opportunity for invasive bacteria to gain entry into the body. This is compounded by the fact that the onset of necrotizing fasciitis may be masked by what appear to be typical postoperative symptoms.

Some Conditions You Should Not Overlook

While you may be vigilant in being on the alert for NF following cuts, scratches, and bruises, many are not aware of a few other conditions that may also pave the way for NF-causing bacteria to enter. If you have any of the following conditions or situations, don't forget that these, too, may serve as gateways for NF-causing bacteria:

- Athlete's foot and other fungal infections
- Cystitis/vaginitis (infections of bladder and vagina)
- Body piercing
- Dermatitis
- Hemorrhoids
- Sunburn or other type of burns

Can One Have a Predisposition to Contracting NF?

Some aspects of how and why NF attacks are still not completely understood by researchers at this time. For example, is there a predisposition to contracting NF? As we've often said, NF-causing bacteria reside all around us, and yet, invasive infections like necrotizing fasciitis are uncommon. Why doesn't NF affect everyone who is exposed to the bacteria? As of this writing, we can only guess. In an article published in the *Salt Lake Tribune* in 1996 about a local NF victim, Dr. Dennis L. Stevens, widely published infectious diseases physician and researcher of necrotizing fasciitis explained, "People who are stricken with necrotizing fasciitis may have some immune system predisposition, but science can't yet identify it." He says, "I don't think we understand the host factors of the disease well enough. We don't have very much information on immunity to group A strep infections of any type. Most of the work has been studying the organism and not nearly as much as studying the host."

Further, a possible predisposition may explain why some people get mild infections while others get life-threatening or deadly infections. In addition to the fact that serotypes have varying degrees of virulence, some people may, for unknown reasons, be more susceptible. This can come from a variety of reasons, including a person's general level of health, speed of diagnosis, treatment rendered, and lack of antibodies.

So while the experts continue to research why some people contract NF while others don't, we believe it is important to make the point that no one appears to be immune to necrotizing fasciitis. It can happen to anyone—young, old, healthy, or unhealthy. All of us need to be aware of the disease, familiar with symptoms, and informed enough to protect our loved ones and ourselves should it ever occur. In Part Two, we will discuss the diagnosis and treatment of necrotizing fasciitis.

PART TWO

Diagnosis and Treatment

As you know by now after reading Part One, NF is a widely misunderstood disease: Even doctors don't completely understand it. As such, the diagnosis is often missed, with tragic results. Here, in Part Two, we will guide you through the process of a proper and timely diagnosis. We'll also discuss the problem of the missed and/or delayed diagnosis and tell you how the disease is treated. Finally we'll wrap up Part Two by reporting on emerging diagnostic tools, treatments, and drugs that will have a monumental impact on the disease—and offer tremendous hope in minimizing the death and destruction caused by necrotizing fasciitis.

(6)

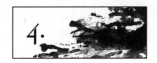

Making the Diagnosis

⑥

THE MEDICAL literature regarding necrotizing fasciitis is quite adamant on this point: *Delay in diagnosis directly results in decreased chances for survival.* In the same breath, however, it must be said that the diagnosis of NF (in the early stages) is a very difficult one to make. In the face of such enormous challenges, how can a physician make a prompt and accurate diagnosis of this deadly disease in time to save the patient and minimize the need for mutilation or amputation? Physicians rely on several distinct but interwoven resources to guide them in diagnosing necrotizing fasciitis: clinical suspicion, the patient's clinical picture (or the symptoms he or she presents), consultations with specialists, exploratory surgery, imaging studies such as the CT scan and MRI, and laboratory tests.

In this chapter we will guide you through the tools and procedures a physician uses in making the diagnosis of necrotizing fasciitis.

Clinical Suspicion: The Physician's Most Powerful Weapon

If a physician is knowledgeable about NF and is paying close attention, there are significant clues in the patient's clinical picture (what a doctor sees upon examining a patient) that can lead to the diagnosis of necrotizing fasciitis. In addition to severe flulike complaints, perhaps one of the most telling symptoms of necrotizing fasciitis is pain out of proportion to the injury. For example, a patient may arrive at the emergency room complaining of flulike symptoms and unbearable pain in a limb or other area of their body. The sensation of pain is a subjective one that a physician cannot measure or quantify. Unfortunately, this may make it less significant in the physician's mind as he or she attempts to make a connection between what the patient reports and what the physician can clinically observe. Accordingly, the doctor may conclude, for example, that the patient may simply have a low tolerance for pain, a pinched nerve, muscle strain, or thrombosis (blood clot) in the limb.

A physician's most powerful weapon in the battle against necrotizing fasciitis is a high level of clinical suspicion. If a physician is suspicious of a necrotizing infection in the earliest stages of NF, a patient's chances for survival are excellent. If the patient is sent home with an incorrect diagnosis (a very common occurrence, as you will read in the next chapter), he or she will inevitably return to the physician within a day or two with advanced symptoms. At that time the swelling, mottled skin, and bullae formation may trigger enough suspicion for the physician to investigate further. Or, tragically enough, the patient may be sent home again. If the patient is allowed to reach critical symptoms and suffer toxic shock, no level of suspicion can make up for the extensive damage done to the patient.

> Although the emergency specialist had not personally experienced a case [of NF] before, he made the diagnosis within ten minutes of examination. The physician relied on the look in my wife's eyes and the resultant tingling he felt in the back of his neck that made his hair stand on end. He calls this his "Spidey sense," [after the comic-book character Spiderman—and it has served him well in his eleven years in emergency medicine]. So much for dry clinical approaches! Because of this "sense," diagnosis and treatment were exemplary. In fact, today we delivered a bottle of champagne and a Spiderman doll to this wonderful physician to thank him.
>
> —Ross Gilley, about his wife, Airlie

The condition of the patient's skin is also an important clue to the diagnosis of NF. In the early stages the skin may appear only slightly swollen and shiny, with an area of reddened, hot skin. When palpitated, the physician may feel what is called *crepitus,* a grating or crackling sound caused by air or gasses in the subcutaneous tissues, although this does not occur in group A strep infections. At this point the physician may suspect an underlying necrotizing soft-tissue infection.

These deciding clues strongly suggest a diagnosis of NF and, if heeded, go a long way to ensure that the patient is treated promptly and aggressively. The suspicion of necrotizing fasciitis, however, is only the beginning. The physician must then confirm the diagnosis. We'll discuss how this is accomplished in the following paragraphs.

The Infectious Disease Specialist

If a physician suspects that a patient is suffering from NF, he or she will seek assistance in confirming the diagnosis through consultation with an infectious disease (ID) physician.

The role of an ID specialist cannot be understated, since the symptoms, manifestation, and treatment of NF are bound to be more familiar to a specialist trained to seek out such infections than to a general-practice physician. The ID specialist also becomes instrumental during treatment by examining the patient regularly; overseeing the use, type, and effectiveness of antibiotics and other treatment options; and monitoring the patient's blood and tissue cultures.

Exploratory Surgery

When a doctor strongly suspects an underlying necrotizing soft-tissue infection, he or she will call upon a general surgeon to perform exploratory surgery to confirm the diagnosis. This may occur immediately if the symptoms are extremely suspicious, or often, may follow certain supportive diagnostic testing, such as those we discuss in this chapter as well as in chapter 7. The exploratory surgery is not a complicated procedure. Essentially the patient is placed under general anesthesia, and the area of the body to be cut is swabbed with an antimicrobial agent. The surgeon then makes an incision in the suspicious area through the subcutaneous tissue down to the fascial layer, which lies directly above the muscle. He or she then closely examines the subcutaneous tissue and fasciae for signs of dead tissue. Unlike normal subcutaneous tissue, dead tissue appears gray or green/yellow and stringy, does not bleed when cut, and is easily separated from the underlying fasciae (a phenomenon known as undermining), while healthy subcutaneous tissue normally adheres to fasciae. Fluid drainage, which the surgeon collects for analysis, may also be present.

If the surgeon discovers any of these conditions, he or she will more than likely expand the surgery to remove the dead tissue—an operation called debridement, which we will discuss in greater detail in Chapter 6—or amputate affected fingers, toes, arms, or legs, if necessary. A plastic surgeon will also step in to handle skin grafting when the patient is well on the road to recovery. (You will learn more about any necessary plastic surgery in Chapter 6.) If, on the other hand, the tissue bleeds normally and appears healthy, it will most likely be determined that the patient is suffering from cellulitis or some other superficial infection.

The decision to perform exploratory surgery to confirm his or her suspicions of necrotizing fasciitis is the most consequential one that a physician can make in the treatment of a patient with NF. While putting a patient "under the knife" is often regarded as a last resort, for NF patients the opposite is true: Even if the patient is considered a poor surgical candidate due to underlying health problems, confirming the diagnosis via exploratory surgery is still a better option than allowing the disease to run its course unabated. Physicians and researchers educated in the course of NF drive this pivotal point home repeatedly throughout the medical literature. For example, in an excellent article entitled "Necrotizing Fasciitis: Don't Wait to Make a Diagnosis," Dennis L. Stevens, M.D., makes a rather emphatic point to his colleagues:

> If primary care physicians are concerned that a deeper infection might be present, surgical evaluation is warranted. Thus, we should have the same general philosophy with soft-tissue infection that we have with appendicitis. It is better to subject some

patients with symptoms mimicking appendicitis to unnecessary surgery than to miss operating on the patient with a ruptured appendix. Failure to diagnose necrotizing fasciitis early may be a fatal mistake.

Imaging Studies

The physician's clinical suspicion, the patient's clinical picture, consultations with specialists, and exploratory surgery are critical to the diagnosis of NF. However, the remaining two resources—imaging studies and laboratory tests—are often used as a means to confirm and clarify the diagnosis after initial consultation and surgery. Generally they are used after surgery because the time it takes to conduct these tests and wait for results is not in the best interests of a patient in the throes of a rapidly progressing necrotizing infection.

CT scans and MRIs are both diagnostic tests that provide physicians with high-resolution pictures of the inside of the body. Both procedures utilize state-of-the-art computerized technology. The equipment for both procedures is quite large, resembling a huge cylinder through which the reclining patient is placed. CT scans and MRIs are highly advanced procedures that can be excellent alternatives to exploratory surgery. In some cases, by using these imaging studies, abnormalities can be detected without subjecting the patient to the risks of surgery.

These imaging studies are effective in detecting soft-tissue inflammation and fluid accumulation. They can also detect the presence of subcutaneous emphysema (the presence of gasses in the subcutaneous tissues), which is a byproduct of infection caused by certain types of bacteria, usually mixed aerobic/anaerobic infections. This knowledge greatly assists the physician in establishing the extent of the infection and in tailoring antibiotic therapy. Necrotizing fasciitis caused by group A strep does not cause subcutaneous emphysema, whereas clostridia, gram-negative bacteria, and *Bacteroides* do. According to Dr. Stevens, the absence of gasses in the subcutaneous tissues may throw the physician completely off the trail by causing him or her to erroneously believe that the patient is suffering from a "benign process."

The CT Scan

The CT scan, or computerized tomography scan, was developed in the early 1970s. It is done with a highly sensitive X-ray beam that is directed on a certain area of the body, such as the abdomen or chest area. Sometimes a type of dye is ingested or injected into the patient to allow greater contrast on the images. As this beam passes through the body it detects an image, and the data are translated into a computer. The computer then analyzes the information and creates an image on a television screen. The image displayed is in the form of a cross-section of the body, giving the radiologist a comprehensive view of what is going on inside the body.

The MRI

Magnetic resonance imaging (MRI) was introduced into mainstream medicine in the late 1980s. This type of diagnostic imaging uses radio waves and huge magnets to create an intensely strong magnetic field. Basically, after the MRI device creates a magnetic field, it sends radio waves into the body that affect hydrogen, an element that exists in each of our cells. Through a sophisticated mapping procedure, which draws on the response of hydrogen to the magnetic waves, the computer creates a three-dimensional picture of the inside of the body. Although the MRI is more expensive than the CT scan, it gives the radiologist a much more detailed view of the body and is highly effective in investigating abnormalities in the brain and central nervous system.

Laboratory Tests

Laboratory tests involve taking a sample of the tissue or blood from the patient and having it analyzed for telltale signs of an underlying infectious process, as well as to determine the species of bacteria that are causing the infection. Lab tests also provide physicians important information regarding the health of major organs, such as the kidneys, heart, and lungs, particularly when the patient is suffering from toxic shock. Lab tests are performed daily and sometimes even more frequently during the patient's treatment until the patient stabilizes.

Laboratory test results in NF patients will show several abnormalities indicative of a severe infection. Typically the patient's number of white blood cells will be much higher than normal, signaling that the body is fighting an infection. Other blood test results may further demonstrate inflammation in the patient's system. A test for creatine phosphokinase, an enzyme present in muscle tissue, may also be elevated in patients with NF, due to tissue breakdown. Furthermore, NF patients often show an increased level of creatinine, a product of creatine, which is associated with abnormal kidney function, a common finding in NF patients.

&

The early signs of a necrotizing soft tissue infection are deceptive. The patient often exhibits precious few physical clues to account for his or her genuine complaints. It is at this early stage—before the bacteria can succeed in flooding the body with toxins—that the prompt and accurate diagnosis of NF needs to be made. But in order for this to happen, a physician must often trust his or her gut instincts and act quickly, decisively, and aggressively to confirm the diagnosis. In order for the suspicion of NF to be raised, a kernel of knowledge about the disease—its symptoms and predisposing conditions—must exist in the physician's mind to begin with. If no knowledge of NF exists, there can be no suspicion and without suspicion, there can be little hope of a prompt and accurate diagnosis. This leads us into the next chapter which investigates the widespread problem of the missed and/or delayed diagnosis of necrotizing fasciitis.

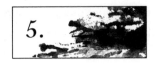

5.

Why Necrotizing Fasciitis Is Often Misdiagnosed

⑥

THIS CHAPTER was very difficult for us to write, as the issue of misdiagnosis and NF is extremely emotional for both the patient and physician—not to mention for us. To explain: as the "clearinghouse" for NF, we at the National Necrotizing Fasciitis Foundation receive calls and e-mails daily from all over the world from people reporting yet another fatal or nearly fatal case of NF that was tragically misdiagnosed. Even though the victims may be thousands of miles apart, the elements of the stories shared with us are consistently similar. There are several reasons for this, as we will explain in this chapter. Having to comfort another grieving parent, spouse, or child of an NF victim who might have lived had the diagnosis been made earlier will never get easier for us. The pursuit of litigation is common. But because we are in a unique position to clearly see a distinct pattern of misdiagnosis of NF across the board among physicians, we feel this chapter is necessary and can help to save lives. We have worked with several physicians in writing this chapter, and we thank them for their candidness, their criticism, and their invaluable perspective as medical professionals who diagnose and treat NF patients in their practices.

In this chapter, we will focus on the high rate of misdiagnosis of necrotizing fasciitis by physicians. We will share the experiences of several NF patients and present an in-depth look into the complex reasons why the diagnosis of NF is often delayed or missed altogether. Such pressing concerns as the similarities between NF's manifestations and the manifestations of other disorders and how the policies of health-maintenance organizations (HMOs) contribute to missed or delayed diagnoses, will be discussed. In addition, we will talk about what is being done to encourage greater awareness and education for not only doctors, but nurses as well, as they play a very important role in recognizing symptoms.

The Prevalence of Misdiagnosis

Since our foundation's inception in early 1997, we (the authors) have been compiling an extensive database of NF cases. In doing so, we have been struck by the number of people who reported to us that when they sought treatment for their symptoms, they were sent home with incorrect diagnoses—sometimes more than once. Despite the attention generated by the disease in recent years in both the medical literature and the media, the trend continues.

> On February 9, 1999, I lost my brother-in-law, Dave, to this disease. As it seems with all the other cases, he, too, started out with flulike symptoms and a sore arm. He was told during his brief sickness to go home, rest, and take Advil. Right up until his last few hours, they [the doctors, specialists] were still puzzled as to what he was suffering from. They continued to treat his arm for blood clots. It is downright scary to look at all of the other cases and see that they are all the same, almost word for word. I am still in disbelief of all the doctors' lack of knowledge that was involved in this tragedy. Dave was 36, and will always be remembered by his beautiful wife, four wonderful children, loving parents and sister, parents-in-law, extended family, and of course his brother-in-law.
>
> —Shawn H.

Misdiagnosis of NF occurs not only in the early stages, when the disease is extremely difficult to identify, but also sometimes in the face of classic, progressing symptoms, such as bullae formation, mottled skin, and toxic shock. Patients have reported being diagnosed erroneously with everything from the flu to arthritis, sprained arms or ankles, pulled muscles, ingrown toenails, hernia, heart attack, yeast infection, broken bones, self-inflicted injury, bursitis, boils, bowel obstruction, aneurysm, etc.

As we begin our discussion of the misdiagnosis problem, it is important to keep in mind that the great majority of the world's physicians are caring human beings who are devoted to saving lives. They would not knowingly send a patient home, undiagnosed and untreated, who is suffering from a deadly disease like necrotizing fasciitis. However, the fact remains that it happens all too frequently, for reasons we will discuss throughout this chapter. While each case is unique in terms of entry point, type of bacteria involved, time elapsed, and ultimate outcome, a general pattern has evolved:

1. The patient exhibits early, progressing symptoms and makes one or more attempts to seek medical treatment, but is sent home with an erroneous diagnoses.
2. His or her condition steadily worsens and becomes critical.
3. The patient is returned to the hospital, where emergency medical intervention is initiated, the effectiveness of which is considerably weakened due to the advanced stage of the disease, which directly results in loss of limbs, permanent disability, severe disfigurement, or death.

Bob Borge, a 46-year-old technician in the California film industry, asked a friend to drive him to the emergency room of a Los Angeles hospital. He had a high fever, nausea, and excruciating pain that seared through his arm and into his shoulder. After waiting several hours to be seen by a physician, Bob was sent home—undiagnosed—with a prescription for pain and his arm in a sling. He returned the following day with worsening symptoms but was again sent home by the plainly annoyed treating physician. The third time he sought care, Bob was deathly ill and begged to be admitted. He lay on a gurney in an examination room in the emergency room alone and screaming in pain with no medical treatment from 9:30 A.M. until 4:30 P.M. When the hospital staff finally looked in on him, they asked him to leave the hospital. "There is nothing wrong with you," they told him. "You're a hypochondriac and a baby."

But Bob was having none of it. He made a scene—demanding loudly for someone to take him seriously—and was harshly warned to be quiet, as the hospital was "trying to treat people who were really sick." Finally, out of pure desperation, Bob threatened to commit suicide if the hospital did not admit him. "I just knew I was dying," Bob told us.

Under California state law, the hospital was forced to admit patients who threatened self-harm, and so it was with some sense of relief that Bob found himself assigned to the psychiatric ward for observation. This rather unorthodox decision on Bob's part undoubtedly saved his life. A psychiatric nurse finally heeded his complaints, diagnostic testing was ordered, a diagnosis of necrotizing fasciitis was made, and appropriate treatment was begun. "I believe that the empathy displayed by this nurse and his fast actions were instrumental in saving my life," Bob told us.

However, the damage caused by the rapid spread of the disease fueled by the delay in diagnosis forced Bob to be hospitalized for over ninety days, forty-two of them in the intensive care unit. He underwent dozens of hyperbaric oxygen chamber treatments and repeated surgeries to remove the destroyed tissue from his body. As of this writing, Bob is very happy to be alive, but is left with over half a million dollars in medical bills and a life marred by severe disfigurement and partial disability.

Bob's story is unusual in that most people don't have to resort to such drastic measures for their physicians to take them seriously. Nevertheless, his experience does hold very important lessons: If you believe you or a loved one are truly sick, you must make yourself heard in any way you can. It could save your life. Bob's story also depicts one physician's painful lesson in the recognition of NF: discovering that the patient he brushed off as a hypochondriac was actually suffering from a deadly infection.

The Reasons Misdiagnoses Are Common

After reading the insets describing Bob's story, as well as others, one can be quick to point fingers at primary-care and/or emergency-room physicians for failing to promptly diagnose and treat an NF patient. When the physician fails to make the proper diagnosis (or consult an infectious-diseases expert) even in the face of "textbook" advanced symptoms such as bullae, mottled skin, high fever, and toxic shock, this is certainly understandable—and powerfully underscores the need for continuing education and awareness for physicians on the subject of necrotizing soft-tissue infections. We'll discuss this more later in the chapter.

And yet the lack of awareness of NF in some physicians, while a serious issue in itself, is only part of the problem. As we've mentioned throughout this book, the missed and/or delayed diagnosis of NF can also be attributed to NF's hallmark ability to wreak its devastating damage on the body with few symptoms to show for it—until the disease has reached the critical stage. A recent article in the *British Columbia Medical Journal*, which featured NF as the focus of the April and May 1999 issues, illustrates this point. The covers of the two journals featured caricatures of a wolf in sheep's clothing—a highly appropriate representation of how NF stealthily invades and attacks the body under the guise of a common, minor affliction. An article in the April issue presented the tragic case of a young woman who sought medical treatment from several different physicians over a period of days for severe ankle pain. Unfortunately, the woman's condition quickly deteriorated, and while en route to another hospital, she died of toxic shock associated with necrotizing fasciitis. Laurence S. Hollands, M.D., author of the article, and the physician who had examined the woman toward the end of her illness, gives us some insight into the physician's perspective as he reflects on the woman's death:

Were there any clues in this presentation that would, in the future, help us discover such a problem sooner? It is clearly very difficult. How many times have we all treated similar patients with musculoskeletal pain, tenosynovitis, or acute arthritides of various kinds? We see presentations like this every day. Thousands come through our emergency rooms and clinics each week. For the most part, no lab work is done and temperatures are not recorded because there seems to be no need.

Here was a case that on the surface seemed the same as the rest, but this young woman died, twelve hours after hospitalization. Could we have prevented that? Can we prevent such deaths from occurring in the future? There are a few things we can learn, a few lessons we can take away. But no matter how vigilant we are, this remains an extremely rare disease, often masked, and rapidly fatal."

Dr. Hollands discussed the misdiagnosis issue further with us for this chapter. His comments no doubt reflect those of many physicians: "When the diagnosis of NF is missed, the physician is as upset as the patient with the result. The disease can be virtually impossible to clinically diagnose in time to save the patient. When it happens to a physician, it is something that comes totally out of left field, and the physician is blindsided."

Dr. Hollands makes another crucial observation that we must keep in mind as we investigate the problem of misdiagnosis. At times the symptoms of NF are so beguiling that *several* physicians examining a single patient can fail to make the connection. We now understand that physician awareness is a problem compounded by the fact that the symptoms of NF are deceiving, but why else would NF be misdiagnosed at such an alarming rate? Perhaps a metaphor used often in the medical community can shed some light on the issue: *"If you hear hoofbeats outside your window, chances are it is a horse and not a zebra."*

In other words, as a general rule, physicians should look to common afflictions as the root of a patient's symptoms, even if those symptoms seem similar to those of a rare or exotic disease. Because this metaphor holds true in most situations, a primary-care or emergency-room physician may naturally reject the possibility of the flesh-eating bacteria as the aberrant "zebra" when examining a patient complaining of "flulike symptoms," fever, and severe limb pain. Accordingly, the physician diagnoses and treats what is believed to be a "horse"—a pulled muscle, strangulated hernia, pinched nerve, or thrombosis.

Thus, dismissing the diagnosis of NF out of hand as the unlikely "zebra," can delay the diagnosis of the disease. Knowing this, it appears at first glance that the solution would be to insist that physicians consider NF consistently in the clinical setting, and that they take steps to rule out the diagnosis in patients exhibiting limb pain, fever, or severe flulike symptoms. But to meet this goal, physicians would be forced to subject thousands of people per day to invasive testing or costly imaging studies. In light of the rarity of the disease—only one to five cases per 100,000 people—these measures become impractical and unnecessary. So where do we draw the line between patients that warrant further diagnostic testing and those who don't?

It's an extremely difficult call to make, and requires further study by experts in the disease. A physician's clinical suspicion and knowledge of the manifestation and course of necrotizing soft-tissue infections remains the backbone of the successful diagnosis and treatment of NF. Moreover, while it may not be feasible for physicians to subject every patient with limb pain, fever, or flulike symptoms to further diagnostic measures, perhaps we can decrease the high rate of misdiagnosis of NF by encouraging physicians to be on alert for patients presenting with the aggregation of symptoms—the combination of extreme pain with fever and flulike symptoms—that may be strongly suggestive of NF.

Patients contacting their doctors by telephone to report symptoms versus their being physically examined can also contribute to the high rate of misdiagnosis of NF. After outpatient surgery, for example, if troubling symptoms arise, the patient is instructed to contact the physician by telephone. As we shared in the last chapter, Carol called her doctor three times with worsening symptoms after her bilateral breast surgery. The doctor in charge of her care, relying solely on the symptoms she described over the telephone, diagnosed Carol first with a virus and then with a reaction to the pain medication—both of which turned out to be horribly inaccurate, forcing the removal of the young woman's breasts.

But the fact is that physicians cannot routinely rely exclusively on a patient's description of his or her symptoms over the telephone to make an accurate diagnosis. A proper diagnosis—which includes ruling out more serious conditions in the differential diagnosis—requires the examination of separate pieces of a diagnostic puzzle that, when assembled, reveals enough information to allow an informed decision to be made. The pieces of the puzzle include subjective symptoms, which are those personally relayed by the patient; where a physician actually examines a patient with his or her own eyes; and supporting data from medical tests

The Differential Diagnosis

The differential diagnosis is defined as the differentiating of a disease or condition from others presenting comparable symptoms. It is a process as fundamental to the practice of medicine as blueprints are to the field of architecture. For example, suppose that a man walks into the emergency room of a hospital complaining of a splitting headache. While the treating ER physician may initially suspect a migraine, he or she has a duty under the differential diagnosis policy to rule out other viable, more serious conditions that could also cause severe head pain.

In order to rule out more serious conditions, the physician develops a running list of possible causes for the man's complaints, and, like a detective narrowing down a field of potential suspects, begins an investigation. This includes taking the patient's history, wherein the physician asks the patient a battery of questions regarding important clues such as allergies, change in vision, unusual work demands, and recent head, neck, or back injuries.

The investigation also includes a thorough physical examination. Blood or urine tests may be ordered, as well as imaging studies such as X rays, MRI, and CT scan. Finally, after carefully weighing all of the information gathered, the doctor makes an intelligent diagnosis, based on sound clinical judgment, diagnostic testing, and the process of elimination.

like blood work, X rays, CT scans, and others. In the absence of any one of these puzzle pieces, the potential for diagnostic errors increases.

In some cases of NF, the potential for misdiagnosis is also heightened when the patient seeks medical attention from more than one physician after the onset of symptoms. In the case described by Dr. Hollands earlier in this chapter, the patient saw five different physicians on five different occasions. While in normal circumstances a second opinion is more beneficial than not, in some NF cases the diagnosis can become lost when more than one physician is consulted.

The Importance of Education in the Medical Community

The need for education and awareness is a predominant theme throughout this book. In many cases, such as those we have described, the diagnosis of NF is tragically missed because of a lack of awareness of the disease, compounded by its extraordinarily furtive and swift course. Knowing this, what is being done to educate the medical community regarding NF?

My nineteen-year-old college freshman son died on March 4, 1998, from NF. On March 2, he developed flulike symptoms and severe pain in his right chest area. He was taken to the emergency room at 5:30 A.M. on March 3. A chest X ray and a CT scan of his lungs were conducted. Both were normal. He was given two shots of Demerol, which did not relieve his pain. He was sent home with anti-inflammatory and pain medications. The diagnosis was flu and a pinched nerve or pulled muscle.

The next afternoon an ambulance was called because he was growing worse. By the time of his arrival at the ER, he had no blood pressure and was dehydrated and in shock. His organs were failing. He was moved to the intensive-care unit, where a team of doctors continued to be baffled by his condition. Only minutes before his death did they make a tentative diagnosis of

NF. They were preparing to do surgery when he went into cardiac arrest and died at 10:40 P.M., eight hours after his admission to the ER. We are still in shock and utter disbelief that this happened to our healthy, vibrant boy.

Within the span of two days a rare disease cut our son down in the prime of his life. The initial misdiagnosis and the failure to diagnose until too late are incomprehensible to us. An autopsy confirmed NF due to strep A bacteria. The germ is thought to have entered his body from a scrape on his elbow and festered in an area of his chest where he had received soft-tissue damage. Nothing was visible on the skin, except for a slight swelling on the right side of his chest.

—Carey Porter

Educating Physicians about NF

At the National Necrotizing Fasciitis Foundation, our goal is to increase knowledge about NF in both the medical and the lay communities. We strive to fill the informational void about NF for doctors by answering direct questions, making referrals, and disseminating information via our Web site, mail, the media, public speaking, and this book. Another organization, Surviving Strep, based in Ontario, Canada, is dedicated to researching and providing education about streptococcal diseases. (See the Resources section of this book for information about this organization.)

Leading infectious disease experts are also hard at work to alert physicians to the problem of misdiagnosis. Alan L. Bisno, M.D., of the Department of Veterans Affairs, and vice chairman of the University of Miami Medical Center, has spearheaded a research project—of which we are honored to be a part—about the misdiagnosis of NF by physicians. Dr. Bisno will be presenting an in-depth analysis of a number of cases of misdiagnosis in an effort to inform the medical community of the dangers of overlooking this uncommon but deadly infection.

Our role has been to compile data from victims or family members regarding their experiences with NF and the manner in which the physicians responded. To accomplish this, we developed a detailed questionnaire and posted it on the NNFF Web site. The responses to these questionnaires were then forwarded to Dr. Bisno for his evaluation and investigation, which included an exhaustive review of the patient's medical records.

Dr. Bisno's findings will be made available to health-care providers in the medical journal *Clinical Infectious Diseases* in late 2000. As medical journals are a premier source of information and continuing education for physicians, we sincerely hope that Dr. Bisno's article will bring the problem of misdiagnosis of NF to the forefront of the medical community.

The Need for Education About Necrotizing Fasciitis Among HMOs

I am a survivor with serious concerns about how doctors and HMOs handle this serious disease [NF]. I had horrible treatment from most of my doctors because they were too involved with gaining the approval of their own group in allowing procedures and investigations of diseases that might require bringing in specialists from outside the area. Diagnosis was delayed for approximately two weeks because of the local doctors' unwillingness to bring a specialist to the area.

—Kathleen

Health maintenance organizations (HMOs) are the subject of much debate at present for reasons that coincide with the missed and/or delayed diagnosis of NF. In light of what we now know about the dire need for prompt diagnosis and aggressive medical treatment for NF patients, this issue becomes critical. Consider the results of a 1995 survey of 1,710 physicians by the National Center for Policy Analysis:

- Nearly two in five physicians (38 percent) report that their ability to make the right decisions for their patients has declined in the past three years.

- Forty-one percent report a decrease in the amount of time they spent with patients over the previous three years.
- Almost half of those in plans that pay providers either a discounted price or a fixed annual amount per patient rate their ability to get necessary treatment for patients—through referrals, for example—as fair or poor, and almost two thirds (62 percent) rate their ability to get immediate approval for care as low.
- Sixty percent report very serious or somewhat serious problems with external review and with limitations on their clinical decisions.

The following experience of "Laura," a homemaker in her early fifties, is an excellent example of the problems encountered by NF victims who are at the mercy of the bottom-line-comes-first policies of some HMOs.

Laura believes that while vacationing in Fiji with her husband, a mosquito bite on her right thigh allowed group A strep to begin its attack. With her leg swelling and severe flulike symptoms, Laura was seen at a hospital in Fiji, where she was given penicillin, aspirin, and Valium.

After surviving the flight home, Laura was immediately taken to a hospital in her hometown. At this point her leg was swollen to twice its normal size and was developing bullae, a sign of advanced NF. She spent several hours at the emergency room with classic, progressive symptoms; however, Laura's primary-care physician could not come up with a diagnosis and told her that he was sending her home.

Incredulous, Laura demanded to be admitted "until someone could tell me what was wrong." She also demanded to be seen by an expert in infectious diseases, but her physician refused to bring in an infectious-disease specialist, as none existed within his HMO. Laura spent a short time in the hospital and was then released on antibiotics.

However, still clueless as to what was causing his wife's illness, Laura's husband, "Simon," again made a request to the physician to approve a consultation with an infectious disease physician. This request was again refused. Seething, Simon contacted the insurance company directly to coerce the HMO to authorize the consultation. His request was granted. Consequently the specialist examined Laura, diagnosed her with NF, and ordered the medical treatment the severity of her condition warranted.

There are too many stories like Laura's. For this reason, legislation to restructure the way HMOs are allowed to conduct business is needed. In addition to other changes being proposed, it is critical that HMOs allow patients to directly consult specialists when necessary. HMOs must also be called upon to cease the practice of rewarding physicians for refusing to make referrals to specialists or to order laboratory or other diagnostic testing for patients who need them.

The Need for Education about NF among Nurses

As the front line of medical treatment, nurses play an invaluable role in recognizing the symptoms of NF. Several NF victims have reported that it was only because of a nurse's sharp observation skills and gut instincts that a diagnosis of NF was made. Consider "Jeannie's" story, for instance.

An elderly woman was admitted for observation to the small midwestern hospital where Jeannie had been employed as a nurse for a number of years. Jeannie noted that the patient's condition was steadily deteriorating. She was unresponsive and her body was swollen with fluid and exuded a foul odor. The treating physician showed little concern, and the only action taken about the offensive odor was a demand by the other nurses on the floor to keep the hospital room door closed! Jeannie found all this rather unsettling. Her patient was dying of something, the family was upset, and no one seemed to be doing anything about it. Jeannie knew she couldn't just stand idly by.

Risking a reprimand from the treating physician, Jeannie took it upon herself to consult a surgeon on staff at the hospital, who agreed to examine the woman. The surgeon made an immediate diagnosis of NF. The source of the foul odor, he discovered, was gangrene, which was so widespread throughout the woman's body that no intervention was possible. The woman died shortly thereafter.

What we can learn from this tragic case is that a nurse must not hesitate to trust his or her own instincts, training, and clinical experience.

Whether the NF patient is seeking medical attention at a busy emergency room or is recovering in the hospital after surgery, the nursing staff can be the key to recognition of symptoms, timely diagnosis, and aggressive treatment.

We have tried throughout this chapter to present the reality of the misdiagnosis problem fairly and candidly for both patients and physicians. Without question, the lack of awareness of NF—or the failure to consider the disease in the differential diagnosis—by primary care and emergency physicians has resulted in repeated misdiagnoses in many patients, causing severe disfigurement or death as in the cases we have discussed herein. Clearly, immediate and ongoing efforts to educate the medical community about this deadly disease are greatly needed to prevent such tragedies from occurring in the future.

It must also be understood, however, that NF is an uncommon disease that is swift, ruthless, and remarkably surreptitious. In the early stages of the disease, the sheer lack of significant symptoms may make it next to impossible to recognize that a severe infectious process is at work. What's more, in cases where NF is complicated by streptococcal toxic shock syndrome (STSS), the speed and deadliness of the disease make it extremely difficult to diagnose and treat in the narrow window of time that would have any significant effect on the patient. For these difficult cases we can only pray that increased awareness combined with the mainstream utilization of emerging diagnostic tools and treatments such those introduced in Chapter 7 of this book, will prove to be successful.

In the next chapter, we will look at the way NF is treated after the diagnosis has been made.

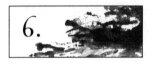

6.

Treating
Necrotizing Fasciitis

⑥

In this chapter we will discuss the wide range of conventional medical treatments that NF patients may receive once the diagnosis is made and the patient is hospitalized. Medical treatment usually consists of several important goals: halting the spread of infection, eradicating the bacteria from the body, salvaging as much viable tissue as possible, protecting the internal organs from permanent damage, and slowly and steadily guiding the patient out of danger and onto the road to healing.

Accomplishing these goals is difficult in and of itself for the medical team; however, in addition, there are many complications, such as organ failure, adult respiratory distress syndrome, and toxic shock, that can arise throughout treatment and cause very serious problems for the patient. We will discuss these complications as well and how they are managed.

Treatments

As you can well imagine from reading this book thus far, the condition of the patient upon admission can vary dramatically, depending upon the stage of the disease. If the disease is caught in its earliest stages, treatment may be limited to debridement, antibiotic therapy, and nutritional support. Accordingly, if the patient is admitted with critical symptoms and/or is of poor underlying health, treatment will be much more involved.

In the most severe cases of NF, patients are admitted to the intensive care unit of the hospital, or at least, to private rooms. As would be the case with any infectious patients, most doctors and nurses don gloves and gowns before handling NF patients. These precautionary measures not only minimize risk to the doctors and nurses but also lessen the risk of secondary infection of the patient.

Let's begin with the most important element of the medical treatment of NF: surgical debridement.

Debridement Surgery

Once a necrotizing soft-tissue infection is confirmed, the dead tissue must be removed. This process is call debridement. While not always possible, ideally this procedure is undertaken when the patient is stabilized. The extent of tissue death can be quite surprising for the surgeon and treating physician, as it is often difficult to estimate how much of the subcutaneous tissue is affected until the patient is inspected internally.

The skin may or may not require surgical debridement. If the overlying skin is free of infection, it is left alone. Other times it is necessary to remove large areas of soft tissue, skin included. The surgeon will continue to cut away until normal, healthy, bleeding tissue is reached.

Following debridement, the wounds are left open to allow for quick inspection. They are treated at bedside.

Patients often require multiple debridements over the course of days or even weeks: Sometimes the procedure must be done as many as thirty or forty times! As the infected tissue can spread from one area of the body to another, even during treatment, it is not unusual for patients to be infected in different areas of the body. In most cases patients will require periodic minor debridement at the bedside throughout their course of therapy. The open wounds are examined and dressed two to three times a day to promote wound healing and help avoid secondary infections so common in the hospital setting.

Without aggressive surgical debridement, all of the other treatments we discuss in this chapter won't make a difference. Debridement is absolutely essential in the treatment of necrotizing fasciitis.

Antibiotic Therapy

Intravenous antibiotic therapy is also a mainstay of the treatment of necrotizing fasciitis. When a case of NF is suspected but not yet confirmed, physicians may order what is known as broad-spectrum antibiotics. This is a cocktail of one or more high-powered drugs designed to be effective against a wide range of bacteria—anaerobic and aerobic— that might be causing the infection. When the laboratory tests reveal the actual culprits, the appropriate drugs can then be tailored accordingly. Penicillin and clindamycin, among others, are antibiotics typically used. Unfortunately, antibiotics will not repair tissue that is already dead or halt the damage of the toxins being exuded, but they will stop the spread of infection.

Induced Sedation

During treatment, many patients are sedated. In the most severe cases the sedation can be prolonged for several weeks. This medically induced relaxation has many benefits, including redirecting the patient's energies to fighting the infection and fighting for survival. It also controls anxiety and pain, which would be a tremendous burden for the patient if he or she were awake. Finally, when it appears that multiple debridements will be required, it makes sense to keep the patient sedated rather than subject him or her to the stress of general anesthesia day after day.

Early in their treatment, many NF patients are cared for in the intensive care unit. They may be on a respirator, and their bodies may be swollen with fluid, a byproduct of the disease and the medical intervention. They may also be surrounded by countless monitors, IVs, and medical equipment. Seeing a loved one in an induced sleep can be quite frightening for family members, although there is some sense of relief that the patient is not awake to experience the terrible pain and discomfort he or she would be subjected to otherwise.

Amputation

Amputation of fingers, toes, limbs, and sometimes breasts and male genitalia is among the most heartbreaking aspects of necrotizing fasciitis. Doctors walk a fine line of trying to save a patient's life and trying not to unnecessarily maim the patient for life. Suffice it to say no surgeon wants to amputate any part of his or her patients' bodies, and the decision is carefully considered within the time constraints forced upon the doctor by the rapid progression of the disease. It is a difficult decision for the physician as well as for the NF victim and family.

Limb ischemia is tissue death in a limb due to restricted blood flow to the area as a result of the toxins produced by the offending bacteria. It is generally the reason for amputation. Limb ischemia can also be attributed to the side effects of the drugs used to treat patients with NF. As you read earlier in this book, one of the symptoms of streptococcal toxic shock syndrome, which often occurs with NF, is dangerously low blood pressure. In order to bring blood pressure back up, drugs like dopamine and norepinephrine are used. These drugs help direct the patient's blood to the vital organs to keep the patient alive, thus taking blood away from the extremities. This can directly cause gangrene of the fingers and toes, necessitating amputation.

The decision to amputate is made to prevent the spread of infection or when it is clear that there is so much tissue death that the limb would no longer be functional. Sometimes the removal of more than one limb may even be necessary. Patients suffering from an underlying health condition such as peripheral vascular disease may be at greater risk for amputation due to the combined insults, as the condition may contribute to the uselessness of the limb or may facilitate the spread of infection. If the patient's condition permits, physicians prefer to conduct the amputation in conservative steps—perhaps removing only a portion of the leg or arm and monitoring it closely. Tissue thought to be viable before one operative procedure may go on to become nonviable during the disease process, requiring further debridement and possible further amputation.

> I'll never forget the phone call. One day, friends of my sister's called to say she was in the hospital with the flu. I was trying to decide whether or not I should go to Michigan to be with her when I got another call. This one completely floored me. It was a doctor saying that my sister had necrotizing fasciitis and that they might have to cut her arm off. In fact, she might die. She was unconscious—not even aware she was ill. I had to make the decision over the phone to say, "Go ahead, do what you need to, cut her arm off if you have to." When I arrived in Michigan, I was relieved to know she had made it out of surgery alive—she was far from out of the woods, but they did not have to cut off her arm. In future days, however, her fingers began to turn black and rot away. They went back in five separate operations to cut off the tip of one finger, then another, and then the majority of a third. I asked the surgeon to be conservative. I begged them to try to bring her out of the medically induced coma so she could make the decision herself. They said they couldn't. So I had to do it. I had to tell them to cut off her fingers. I was afraid she would be angry. She always had beautiful nails and took great pride in her appearance. It broke my heart to have to do it. One of the nurses suggested taking pictures. She said it might help if my sister doubted the necessity of the action. So we took pictures of her black, shriveled up fingers. Thank God that's where the infection stopped. She lost only arm tissue and parts of three fingers. Today she is healthy and happy, and she was not upset at all that I had to make that decision. What a relief.
>
> —Judy, sister of coauthor Donna Batdorff

Bedside care of amputated limbs is undertaken in much the same way as is care of a debrided area of the body—with frequent, sterile dressing changes and close monitoring to watch for secondary infection.

*H*yperbaric *O*xygen *T*herapy *(HBOT)*

Some physicians advocate the use of hyperbaric oxygen (HBO) chambers for the treatment of patients suffering with necrotizing fasciitis due to a mixed anaerobic/aerobic infection, particularly one involving clostridium. However, as of this writing little has been published in the medical literature about the effectiveness of HBO in NF cases, particularly NF caused by group A strep.

What effect does breathing pressurized 100-percent oxygen have on a patient suffering from necrotizing fasciitis? Simply put, the HBO jump-starts the patient's ability to fight infection by flooding the cells with a powerful concentration of oxygen. Provided that there is a viable vascular network extending into the infected tissues, the body's ability to fight infection and promote wound healing is reportedly greatly enhanced by HBOT.

Another important feature of HBO is that pure oxygen destroys anaerobic bacteria—those microorganisms that thrive in the absence of oxygen—diminishing the ferocity of the infectious process. This is the reason that it is widely used to treat gas gangrene, a condition most often caused by anaerobic bacteria. Furthermore, HBOT is useful in helping the surgeon differentiate healthy tissue from infected tissue that must be removed.

Finally, the hyperbaric oxygen chamber is very useful in preparing a patient's tissues for skin graft or skin flap surgery, a procedure in which a section of skin and tissue with the blood supply intact is removed from one area of the body and affixed to another, usually adjacent, area. Oxygenated tissues are healthier and more receptive to the transplant, reducing the risk of skin graft rejection.

In general the HBO chamber consists of an enclosed cylinder with a variety of sophisticated controls operated and continuously monitored by skilled nurses and/or technicians. The reclining patient is placed within the chamber, and the hatchlike door is closed and locked. One-hundred-percent pure oxygen is then pumped into the airtight chamber (the air we generally breathe is only 21-percent oxygen). The chamber is then pressurized according to the nature of the patient's problem. Average atmospheric pressure at sea level is 14.7 pounds per square inch (psi), or 1.0 atmospheres absolute—a unit of measure when discussing high pressure. So, for example, for the treatment of NF, a pressure of 2.0 atmospheres absolute is utilized, which equates to a depth of fifty feet below sea level. The patient remains within the chamber for up to ninety minutes, sometimes as often as three times per day, depending upon the nature of the condition. For NF patients, some physicians believe that HBOT should be used hand in hand with debridement surgery and is most effective when initiated immediately after the first radical debridement and continued throughout the hospital stay, as required for wound healing.

Vacuum-Assisted Closure

A system called vacuum-assisted closure (VAC) has been receiving excellent reviews from physicians in wound management. The system, which utilizes a type of vacuum that uses negative pressure to aid in wound closure and the removal of fluids, can aid healing. VAC can be used as early as the first debridement surgery. A recent study reveals that of 300 wounds treated with the VAC system, 296 responded favorably. Dr. Dennis C. Hammond, in Grand Rapids, Michigan, tells us that he and his staff have been using VAC successfully for about a year and reports that it is a valuable adjunct used in treating difficult open wounds, including those caused by NF.

Complications That Can Arise during Treatment

As we mentioned, many complications can arise during the treatment of necrotizing fasciitis, each of which can be as potentially life threatening as the infection itself. For instance, as previously stated, drugs used for the treatment of low blood pressure may cause tissue ischemia, resulting in the amputation of fingers and toes. Multiple system organ failure, most frequently of the kidneys and lungs, is another complication that can go hand in hand with more virulent strains of bacteria. Organ failure can occur very quickly and can be fatal in many cases.

Adult Respiratory Distress Syndrome

Adult respiratory distress syndrome (ARDS) is another potentially life-threatening complication of NF that results from fluid-filled lungs—a part of overall toxemia. NF patients with ARDS are in extremely critical condition and require breathing assistance with a ventilator. ARDS must be diagnosed quickly, as prolonged lack of oxygen to vital organs can cause permanent damage. Sometimes patients with ARDS are treated with steroids, but the most effective treatment is to aggressively manage the underlying cause of the syndrome.

Lymphedema

Lymphedema is swelling that results when normal drainage of lymph back into the blood is prevented. This can be another unfortunate complication of NF due to damage that infection, surgery, or amputation may cause to the lymphatic system. Permanent damage to the lymphatic system, including the removal of lymph nodes (which fight infection and filter the lymphatic fluid), can cause such effects of lymphedema as severe limb swelling, scar tissue development, and chronic infections such as cellulitis.

Lymphedema is treated in a variety of ways, sometimes with the assistance of a lymphedema therapist. Treatment includes the use of compression garments, pumps to improve the flow of lymph, massage, and various medications.

Systemic Yeast Overgrowth

The long-term use of antibiotics can lead to an overgrowth of yeast in the body, resulting in many debilitating health problems that can frustrate patients as they struggle to regain their health and stamina following a bout with necrotizing fasciitis. Systemic yeast overgrowth can manifest itself in a diverse number of ways, including gastrointestinal upset, fatigue, mood swings, poor memory, asthma, numbness, burning eyes, and many others.

Physicians do not always think of systemic yeast as the possible cause for a person's complaints, and so a patient should not hesitate to bring the possibility of systemic yeast overgrowth to his or her doctor's attention. Systemic yeast must be treated aggressively with antifungal medication.

Secondary Infection

NF patients are prone to secondary infections while hospitalized or during the weeks after being released from the hospital. This may require another hospital stay for constant monitoring and the administration of intravenous antibiotics. Open wounds, as we know, are plentiful opportunities for infections, necrotizing or otherwise, especially when the immune system is severely weakened. For this reason it is very important to take all prescribed antibiotics, pay close attention to your nutritional needs, and pay the utmost attention cleanliness during dressing changes to prevent secondary infections.

Bedsores and Circulation Problems

Bedsores and circulation problems are also troublesome for NF patients, due to the extended period of immobilization they must endure. For both problems there are special devices that can ease pain and discomfort. To help alleviate bedsores, mattresses have been developed that simulate slight movement, repositioning the body every so often while the patient is restrained to the hospital bed. To treat circulation problems, soft air pillows are put around the legs that pump up with air every so often, simulating movement, which aids in circulation.

ICU Psychosis

Another unfortunate complication of long-term hospital confinement and the massive quantities of necessary drugs is a condition known as ICU psychosis. As many as 30 percent of intensive care patients are reported to experience this phenomenon. Patients suffering from ICU psychosis experience hallucinations and are often unable to differentiate between dreams and reality, which can be extremely frightening for the patient as well as loved ones. One gentleman suffering from NF mistook medical equipment for a Native American in full headdress and begged for the hospital staff to make him leave. ICU psychosis is often treated with medication such as Haldol (haloperidol).

Addiction to Painkillers

Addiction to painkillers is another troublesome complication that can arise during the treatment of necrotizing fasciitis. NF patients suffer from excruciating levels of pain, which physicians treat appropriately with drugs such as morphine, Demerol (meperidine hydrochloride), and other potent narcotics. However, while these drugs are blessings to the suffering person, they are highly addictive, and coming off them can be very difficult, both mentally and physically. Symptoms of withdrawals include, but are not limited to, irritability, vomiting, headache, gastrointestinal problems, shaking, and sweating.

Problems Associated with Damaged Skin

Areas of damaged skin can cause permanent annoying problems that must take some getting used to. These include loss of sweat glands, numbness, itching, and sensitivity to sunlight. These complications interfere with many activities including sunbathing, outdoor activities, wearing certain kinds of clothes, and sex. While itching may subside and some sensation may return after several months, or even years, sensitivity to sunlight and numbness are likely to be permanent.

Hair Loss

As if the NF patient doesn't endure enough misery, he or she might also suffer from hair loss as a result of the disease to add insult to injury. This is thought to be caused by the stress caused by NF, medications used to treat it, or a combination of both. The good news is that hair loss as a result of NF is most often temporary. Proper nutrition may be somewhat helpful for preventing this side effect.

⑥

The complications that can arise during an NF patient's treatment are not limited to those discussed here. The road to physical recovery after NF is a bumpy one consisting of good and bad days, with the potential for minor setbacks and unexpected complications, both temporary and permanent. It is critical that all stakeholders in the NF patient's medical care—the many physicians, specialists, nurses, and family members—be constantly on alert and in continuous communication with each other regarding the complicated course of treatment.

Plastic Surgery

Plastic surgeons are the miracle workers that put the NF victim together again after he or she has been ravaged by the bacteria. They play a very important role alongside the surgeon and infectious-disease physician in treating an NF patient. The plastic surgeon should be involved as early in the diagnosis process as possible—i.e., he or she should be present for the first debridement—and remain involved through the daily wound care and subsequent debridements. This prepares him or her for the ensuing reconstructive process that may take place months after the individual is released from the hospital. After all of the debridement surgeries are complete, and it is determined that the patient is free of the bacteria, the plastic surgeon takes over and works the magic of reconstructing the patient's appearance, using such procedures as skin grafts and muscle or skin flaps to close the remaining gaping wounds.

Skin Grafts

Skin grafting involves harvesting viable, healthy skin from one part of the body to use on another area of the body. Often the fronts of the thighs or the buttocks are the most ideal sites to graft the skin from. In order for skin grafting to be successful, the recipient site, or the area the skin is being moved to, must have a healthy blood and nutrient supply.

The skin is harvested in thin strips about three inches wide and approximately one-hundredth of an inch thick, using an instrument known as a dermatome. In the operating room, the harvested skin can also be run through a device that is very much like a pasta machine, which cuts tiny slits into the grafted skin. These cuts cause the skin to expand, allowing it cover a much larger area. This process can be repeated a number of times, making the skin almost double in size. This is useful when a patient has a large wound to cover and not enough skin to cover it.

The harvested skin is then carefully replaced onto the needed areas. Initially nutrients reach the transplanted tissue through the process of osmosis from the recipient site to the transplanted tissue, but within forty-eight hours or so, permanent blood vessels begin to grow into the grafted area. The skin is then stapled or sewn on the open wound in a more permanent fashion, in a complicated process that doesn't always work. Skin grafts can be rejected and need to be treated with the most careful dressing changes and care until it is certain that they have "taken."

Skin Flaps

When the area requiring skin grafting has a poor blood supply, and the chances of rejection are high, surgeons may perform skin flap surgery instead. A skin flap is a section of skin and soft tissue with the blood vessels intact, taken from a healthy area of the body and moved to an adjacent area and affixed. Like skin grafting, a permanent blood supply develops in the new area, allowing the original vessels to be severed. Free flaps are another type of skin flap in which a section of skin and tissue is taken from a more distant location, with the blood supply (arteries and veins) sewn to those at the new location using microsurgical techniques.

Tissue Expansion

Tissue expansion is another method of covering an open wound. It involves actually stretching the skin in the area of the damage. This is accomplished by inserting a balloon-type apparatus under the skin adjacent to the area to be covered. Over several months the balloon is gently expanded, causing the skin to stretch in a manner similar to the way a person's skin stretches with changes like weight gain or pregnancy. In fact, this method causes new skin tissue to actually reproduce, and while the new tissue will not be as thick as the original tissue, it usually contains an excellent blood supply. Tissue expansion also avoids the discoloration and unsightly scars that are an unfortunate side effect of skin grafts or flaps.

Some drawbacks of using tissue expansion include the fact that it is not beneficial for areas of the body that require thicker skin, such as the back. Moreover, the process of tissue expansion can take months, during which time the patient must live with a large balloon bulging from under his or her skin. Overall, the process favors children, women, and the elderly, who have thinner skin. It also appears to be most effective with Caucasians.

The Role of the Family in the Treatment and Recovery of NF Patients

When someone you love is stricken with NF and is barely clinging to life, it is understandable to feel helpless and useless. But you don't have to feel that way: There are ways you can help, even if you have no medical training. Following are some practical suggestions, many of which were contributed by survivors and family members of NF patients, for helping family members contribute to their loved ones' care.

Educate yourself regarding treatment options, and don't hesitate to talk to your loved one's physicians regarding their decisions. Bring resources such as this book to his or her attention, and ask that all options be considered. Keep an open line of communication between you and the physicians and nursing staff. If you are concerned, do not hesitate to make your feelings known. Most physicians are agreeable to discussing patient care with family members; however, if you are not happy with the answers you are receiving, keep asking until you are satisfied.

If the patient is transferred to another, more distant, hospital, find out about resources in the area that may provide a place for the family to stay at a minimal cost. Such places may include hotels with special rates through an arrangement with the hospital, the Ronald McDonald House, etc. The social services department of the hospital is a good place to start asking.

Become part of the health care team by offering to assist in wound care and monitoring the patient. The hospital staff is aware that you are frightfully worried and that participating in patient care in small ways is a welcome change from pacing the floor.

Keeping a daily diary of your loved one's progress may be helpful for the patient, particularly if he or she is unconscious or is a young child. Documenting daily trials and tribulations, how you feel, and what has been going on in your family life will become important to the NF patient as he or she heals and wants to understand exactly what he or she overcame.

Be conscious of illnesses in the family that might be a threat to the recovering NF patient. Maintain a high level of cleanliness around him or her, and ask that young children or sick people refrain from visiting until the patient is clearly "out of the woods."

If the patient is sedated, continue to talk to him or her. There is little scientific evidence to support the notion that your loved one knows you're there, but there is enough anecdotal evidence to believe it is a possibility. One NF patient, an elderly gentleman, would suffer from periodic but severe drops in blood pressure during his struggle with NF. His many nieces and nephews, who were like his own children, never left his side. Despite the fact that the man was in an induced sleep, when his pressure fell, his family members would hold his hands and remind him of the wonderful times that they shared camping at the lake or at family celebrations. To the delight of his family, the man's blood pressure would always rise as a result.

Lastly, never forget that the power of prayer cannot be underestimated! Many people attribute their survival of NF to God and the love of their family.

In this chapter we have explained the mainstays of the treatment of necrotizing fasciitis, namely, surgical debridement, antibiotic therapy, hyperbaric oxygen treatments, and amputation. Only about two-thirds of patients will survive, regardless of how heroic the medical teams' efforts may have been. This is due to the severity of the infection, complications that may arise during treatment, severe infections caught too late, and poor underlying health of the patients. Those who do survive face life as amputees or with tremendous scars, both physical and psychological.

Is this the way it has to be? Is there any cutting-edge technology on the horizon to assist physicians in diagnosing the disease earlier so that lives are saved and mutilation less drastic? Can we ever hope for a miracle drug—a vaccine perhaps—to protect us from contracting the disease in the first place? The answer to both questions is a resounding *"yes!"* God willing, we may beat the disease yet! In the next chapter we'll introduce you to some leading researchers with extremely exciting news about emerging diagnostic tools, treatments, and drugs in the battle against necrotizing fasciitis.

7.

Emerging Diagnostic Tools, Treatments, and Preventive Measures for Necrotizing Fasciitis

(6)

My mom, Jeanne Herrington, passed away on June eighteenth of 1998 after sixty-two days in the hospital with necrotizing fasciitis. She fought very hard to survive! She was an incredibly strong woman, but not strong enough to survive this horrible disease. She had toxic shock syndrome, which destroyed all of her vital organs. I miss her every day of my life and still ask "Why?" It all happened so fast—within a matter of a few hours—from the dental procedure during which she contracted the bacteria to her being on life support. Dear God, help these professionals find a cure and increase the odds of survival. Give those of us in grief some peace with the passing of our dear ones.

—Jan Simonds Hornback

Just because necrotizing fasciitis has beaten us so often in the past and continues to frustrate us in the present does not mean that the future is hopeless when it comes to this killer. On the contrary, as of this writing, there are teams of dedicated researchers, physicians, private organizations, government agencies, and universities working in concert to develop ways to combat NF and other invasive infections.

The information we share in this chapter is exciting, indeed. We will describe emerging tools that are showing great promise in making earlier, more accurate diagnoses of necrotizing soft-tissue infections. Then we will cover innovative treatments that are saving the lives of NF patients once the diagnosis is made. Finally, we'll introduce two landmark vaccines currently in development, as well as a streptococcal-destroying enzyme—all of which will certainly have an historic impact on the prevention of invasive group A strep infections throughout the world.

The Capsular Reactive Protein (CRP) Laboratory Test

Surprisingly, a simple, fast, and inexpensive blood test may provide the "smoking gun" a physician needs to diagnose and confirm a case of NF. Known as the capsular reactive protein (CRP) assay, this blood test measures the amount of CRP in the blood, a substance that is rapidly synthesized in the liver in response to severe bacterial infections such as necrotizing fasciitis.

The normal range of CRP levels in the human body is usually extremely low, or even nondetectable. However, in a patient suffering from a severe bacterial infection such as NF, the level of CRP in the body skyrockets—clearly and consistently indicating a severe infection.

Dr. Rene Chongkit, M.D., a pathologist at Surrey Memorial Hospital, British Columbia, explains, "Should a patient present with flulike symptoms and severe pain out of proportion to the injury and physical findings, the physician may suspect NF or other severe bacterial infection. A request for a CRP assay should be ordered." Within only thirty minutes to an hour, the result of the test will indicate that either the patient's level of CRP is normal (no infection) or elevated (severe infection). Extremely elevated results commonly indicate NF and other severe infections. Therefore, this test serves as objective evidence of the physician's suspicions—leading to swift diagnosis and treatment.

While the CRP test has been in existence for many years, it was previously considered cumbersome and less effective than other laboratory tests in light of the fact that is required twenty-four hours for semi-quantitative results. But because of advancement in technology, CRP testing has evolved to be rapid, repeatable, and dependable.

"However, CRP among physicians in general is still under-utilized," explains Dr. Chongkit, who has performed extensive research into the effectiveness of CRP. "If a physician suspects a serious infection, he or she should perform a CRP assay. If the resulting levels are high, it can be indicative of a serious bacterial infection, the cause of which must be investigated."

CRP testing is also effective throughout an individual's treatment to ensure that a patient's infection is under control. Dramatic drops in CRP levels after treatment are very positive of a resolving infection. However, if CRP levels remain high, the physician should be on alert for continued infection.

Frozen-Tissue Biopsy

Frozen-tissue biopsy in the diagnosis of NF is a simple and quick procedure that is performed at the bedside. Very simply, under local anesthesia, a scoop or "punch" of skin and subcutaneous tissue is removed from the suspicious area. The tissue is then transferred to the laboratory, where it is immediately frozen with liquid nitrogen. The pathologist is then able to conduct several tests on the sample, such as gram-staining, in which a stain is applied to the specimen to identify the type of bacteria involved. By observing how the sample holds the stain, the pathologist can narrow down the type of bacteria involved, such as gram-positive (bacteria that maintain the stain when applied) or gram-negative (those that do not). The pathologist is also able to examine the specimen microscopically for necrotic tissue, thereby making a definitive diagnosis of NF in approximately fifteen minutes from first receiving the tissue biopsy. Frozen-tissue biopsy is not only quick and accurate in the rapid diagnosis of NF, but the risk to the patient is minimal.

Frozen-tissue biopsy can be of tremendous advantage to physicians who suspect a diagnosis of NF but are wavering between a "wait-and-see" approach and exploratory surgery. This diagnostic procedure can be the deciding factor for physicians looking for supportive evidence of their clinical suspicions before operating on the patient.

Intravenous Immunoglobulin

Intravenous immunoglobulin (IVIG) is gaining ever-increasing prominence in the battle against invasive bacterial infections, including NF complicated by toxic shock syndrome. It is already used widely in the treatment of certain AIDS-related conditions, leukemia, chronic fatigue syndrome, cystic fibrosis, and many others.

IVIG is a sterile solution of plasma harvested from a pool of human blood donations. The theory is that plasma is taken from many different people will contain some natural antibodies to various toxins and bacteria that could be a tremendous help to the recipient, who may be lacking the antibodies to fight the infection. The solution floods the bloodstream of the patient with a myriad of nonspecific antibodies, powerfully reinforcing the patient's immune system and, subsequently, the ability to fight off infection.

Dr. Donald Low, based in Toronto and one of Canada's leading researchers of invasive group A strep infrections, published an article in April of 1999 in *Clinical Infectious Diseases* that announced extremely encouraging news regarding the use of intravenous immunoglobulin therapy in patients with flesh-eating disease. Dr. Low noted that the survival rate of NF patients treated with IVIG doubled when compared to a similar group of individuals who were not treated with IVIG. According to one report, the premier of Quebec, Lucien Bouchard, survived his near-death experience with NF due to being treated with IVIG therapy. Unfortunately, this therapy is in short supply, very expensive, and often selectively excluded from insurance coverage.

Group A Strep Vaccines

We are extraordinarily pleased to report that the next five to ten years will see the advent of two historic vaccines that will have the capability of actually preventing infections caused by group A strep. These vaccines are currently being developed separately under the direction of two of the United States' most prominent researchers in group A strep, Dr. James Dale of the University of Tennessee and Dr. Vincent Fischetti of Rockefeller University, New York.

Research has shown that there are more than 100 strains of group A streptococci, many of which are closely related. When a child or adult is infected by a particular strain, he or she develops immunity only to that strain and any closely related strain. This immunity is directed to the M protein, the most abundant protein on the surface of the group A strep bacteria.

Researchers have also determined that the M protein is both good and bad in terms of immunity. On the good side, immunity to the terminal section of the M protein gives protection against subsequent infection, but on the bad side, immunity to the middle of the M protein or conserved section can cause rheumatic fever. This occurs when antibodies developed by the immune system against group A strep also attack human tissues.

Approximately twenty years ago, the U.S. Food and Drug Administration (FDA) banned the use in humans of products containing group A strep after a vaccine trial using a killed whole-cell group A strep vaccine suggested that the vaccine could cause people to produce antibodies that cross-react with human tissues, notably heart tissue (potentially causing rheumatic fever).

The research group at the University of Tennessee and the VA Hospital in Memphis has been working to develop a vaccine against group A strep infections for more than thirty years. The work is currently under the direction of Dr. James Dale, who is optimistic that an effective vaccine can be produced in five to six years.

Their strategy focuses on the important role that the streptococcal M protein plays in these infections, and also on its role in eliciting antibodies that protect against infections. Many studies have shown that an individual who is infected with one serotype of group A strep develops an immune response against that particular type and is not reinfected. Dr. Dale's research group has identified the precise regions of the M protein needed to produce protective immunity in humans. Because each M protein has a different structure, it has been necessary to include pieces of the M protein from many different stereotypes of streptococci.

Using modern biotechnology, Dr. Dale and his research team separated the terminal (or "good") section from the conserved (or "bad") portion, and were able to show in an animal study that if only the good portion was used, the animals developed antibodies which protected them from subsequent infection. When tested on human tissues, these antibodies did not attach, and therefore could not cause rheumatic fever.

In June of 1999, ID Biomedical and its collaborators, the National Institute of Allergy and Infectious Disease (NIAID) and Dr. James Dale at the University of Tennessee, overcame the FDA ban on human testing of products containing group A strep. They are currently conducting a Phase I Clinical Trial sponsored and funded by the NIAID at the University of Maryland's Center for Vaccine Development. Results from the 50-microgram segment of the Phase I study show that at this dose there is no toxicity and no cross-reactive antibodies to human tissues. Although safety is the primary endpoint of the study, all of the volunteers that received the vaccine, even at this low dose, developed antibodies to the six strains targeted by the vaccine.

ID Biomedical and Dr. Dale are currently developing StreptAvax™ for pediatric usage in the developed world, for the prevention of throat infections and invasive infections. The prototypic vaccine, which is currently in a multi-dose Phase I Clinical Trial, covers six strains of group A strep. The product they expect to take into a Phase I/II Clinical Trial later this year will cover an additional 18 prevalent strains of group A strep. The 24-strain vaccine is made from the same technology and manufacturing process as the six-strain product. The final StreptAvax™ formulation is estimated to cover greater than 90 percent of pharyngitis and greater than 95 percent of invasive disease in North America, as well as covering all strains known to cause rheumatic fever (which will be important to India, Africa and several third-world countries).

As of this writing, the University of Maryland's Center for Vaccine

Development is recruiting volunteers for the second arm of the study, in which 100 micrograms of StrepAvax™ will be tested. The vaccine will be injected into the subjects' arms, and their blood will be analyzed to study the antibodies, which are stimulated by the vaccine. If the vaccine is proven to be safe and effective in these early studies, expanded human studies could pave the way for a childhood vaccine that would prevent most group A strep infections and their complications.

Dr. Vincent Fischetti of Rockefeller University in New York is also developing a vaccine that would prevent group A streptococcal infections of the throat. If such a vaccine were successful, not only would the number of strep throat infections be drastically reduced, but there would be a substantial impact on serious complications of group A streptococci such as rheumatic fever and rheumatic heart disease. Because the human pharynx is one of the most prevalent places where these organisms are found in the environment, eliminating them from this site will have a significant impact on streptococcal-related diseases in general, such as strep throat and otitis media.

While the vaccine will not benefit patients already suffering from group A streptococcal infections, it will be effective in preventing streptococci from being harbored in the throat in the first place. Very simply, Dr. Fischetti explains, the vaccine works by triggering the body's natural immune responses in serum and saliva to a common region of the M protein which is present on all of the more than 150 different types of M protein found on streptococci. This immune response prevents streptococcal infection by blocking the ability of streptococci to attach to and infect the pharyngeal cells in the oral cavity. Thus the vaccine will prevent infection at its earliest stages. By blocking the ability of these organisms to attach to and infect the pharynx, their ability to be spread to other individuals in respiratory droplets via breath, coughing, and sneezing would be markedly reduced or eliminated.

This vaccine is based on the conserved region of the M protein, which has been implicated in the development of rheumatic fever and therefore must be proved safe before the FDA will allow it to be tested in humans.

The vaccine will be one of the first orally and nasally administered vaccines for the prevention of a bacterial infection. Based on current results, it is anticipated that once this vaccine is tested in humans, it will take another five to six years of human testing before final approval and market release. For more information on this vaccine, we have provided Dr. Fischetti's contact information in the Resources section in this book.

Group A Streptococcal-Destroying Enzyme

Dr. Fischetti is also hard at work on another very promising approach to prevent group A strep infections: an enzyme that actually kills the bacteria within seconds. It accomplishes this by targeting the streptococcal cell wall and destroying the bacteria on contact.

Like the vaccine that Dr. Fischetti is also developing, the enzyme will prevent throat infection at its earliest stages, at the time when the streptococcus first enters the oral cavity. It is envisioned that the enzyme will be administered in the form of a spray or lozenge. Taken when contact with the bacteria is made or anticipated, it will kill the incoming streptococci, thus preventing them from establishing an infection. Such a development would also benefit the one in five adults and children who at any given time carry group A streptococci in their throats without symptoms, preventing those bacteria from actually causing infection. It would also be of value for school-age children, preventing the transmission of streptococci between children in schools and day-care centers and infected siblings in the same household. For health-care workers and others, use of the enzyme will protect them from streptococcal infection and passage of the organism to others.

The advantage of using the enzyme over an antibiotic is that the enzyme kills only the group A streptococcal bacteria and not the healthy bacteria found in the oral cavity. The enzyme is currently under development and should be available to the public by the end of 2000.

❧

Establishing a powerful arsenal of diagnostic tools, treatments, and preventive medicines, combined with universal knowledge of the symptoms and manifestations of NF by treating physicians, is our best chance at minimizing the rate of tissue destruction and death currently being wrought worldwide by NF-causing bacteria. Accordingly, Dr. Fischetti's and Dr. Dale's respective vaccines will prove to be the most historic advances of the new millennium in the battle against diseases caused by streptococcus. The impact these vaccines will have on the worldwide population is simply mind-boggling. In only a few short years it is quite possible that we will be able to prevent millions of common strep throat infections and their more serious complications in adults and children, as well as invasive group A strep infections, such as necrotizing fasciitis and streptococcal toxic shock syndrome.

PART THREE

⑥

Life After NF

Picking up the pieces of our lives after surviving NF—or going on after we have lost someone we love—requires tremendous strength, courage, faith, and love. In Part Three we will guide you through the multifaceted process of physical, emotional, and spiritual healing. Finally, we will focus on what you can do to promote prevention and awareness in the home, the community, and the workplace.

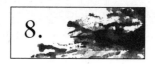

8.

One Woman's Story

❦

$\mathbf{W}$HAT BETTER way to depict the entire experience of surviving necrotizing fasciitis than to tell you the story of a survivor? Cassi Moore is a vibrant, active mother of two. She and her husband, Dan, live in California and enjoy normal, healthy lives. What happened to Cassi, as we have pointed out over and over again, can happen to anyone. It is Cassi's wish that by sharing the intimate details of her story, she will be able to educate others, increase awareness, and perhaps save lives.

❦

On the weekend of June 20 and 21, 1998, Cassi Moore and her three children attended a camp-out with their tae kwon do school. Sometime over the weekend, Cassi sustained a very small cut on her left thumb. She cannot recall how she cut herself but remembers washing the cut and applying antibiotic ointment and a Band-Aid. When practicing defensive tactics, she sustained slight trauma on the left side of her rib cage—either a bruise or a pulled muscle.

She returned home on the morning of the twenty-first and felt very tired and sore. On the morning of the twenty-second she awoke feeling the same way, but her left side hurt as well. By that afternoon she became quite ill. The symptoms included vomiting, diarrhea, a fever, and pain in her side. She was taken to the doctor by her brother and returned home after being diagnosed with the flu and a possible pulled muscle on her left side.

On June 23, Cassi continued to feel ill and also began complaining of severe pain on the upper left side of her rib cage. She returned to the doctor, who prescribed medication for what appeared to be a faint bruise that had appeared on her left side. By that evening the bruised area became very large and was very dark in color.

On the morning of June 24, just three days after her first mild symptoms, Cassi was very weak and needed assistance to get out of bed. She could not breathe well and had trouble seeing. By 11 A.M. the bruise on her side began to ulcerate and leak fluid and blood. By 1 P.M. Cassi, who by now couldn't walk unassisted or see, was taken to the emergency room at an area hospital.

When Cassi arrived at the hospital, her family practitioner was waiting for her. She had no detectable blood pressure and was in septic shock. Her doctor immediately consulted with a surgeon and an infectious disease specialist. They decided to perform a CAT scan on Cassi's side. The scan revealed the necrotizing fasciitis. Cassi was then rushed into the operating room for emergency surgery. During the surgery they removed a large portion of flesh from the left side of her rib cage and part of her breast. Approximately 6 to 8 percent of her body's surface was removed.

After surgery Cassi was moved to the intensive care unit (ICU), where she was placed on a ventilator and vasoconstricting drugs, or "pressers." Pressers are used to artificially elevate the blood pressure when a patient is unable to maintain their own. They work by constricting the blood vessels in the extremities, thereby forcing the blood into the trunk of the body to supply the brain and vital organs. An unfortunate side effect of these drugs is that under prolonged use, the extremities, such as fingers and toes, can suffer damage due to the lack of blood flow.

The wound on her side following surgery had to be left open for a couple of reasons. First, most likely there would have to be additional surgeries to remove further necrosis. The second reason was that a wound that size would have to be covered by a skin graft and first needed to begin granulating, or healing from the inside.

The first night in the intensive care unit was very rough for Cassi and the whole family. She was fully conscious; however, due to her precarious condition and the possibility of additional surgeries, her ventilator tube could not be removed. She also began having pain in her fingers on her right hand. The family began praying in earnest for her survival and for the time when she would no longer need the vasoconstricting drugs, which were beginning to do damage to her hands and feet.

By the morning of June 25, Cassi was unconscious, and the doctors were concerned that she was soon going to require hemodialysis, and since they did not have the capability on-site, they recommended transferring her to another hospital. They feared that she would soon be too unstable to attempt transferring. That afternoon she was transferred, where the attending physician in charge of the intensive care unit did not give the family much hope for her survival. He immediately made arrangements for her to be airlifted to a San Francisco local medical center, where she would wage a battle for her life over the next three weeks. Her family set up camp in the waiting room and never left her side during the entire ordeal.

During the first few days the family began to have hope that Cassi would survive; however, it also became apparent that her hands and feet would be seriously damaged. Cassi's fingers, toes, and parts of her right foot began to turn first purple and then black. Still, there was hope that even this would be reversed, until on the third and fourth days, her fingers and toes began to shrivel. She also required hemodialysis treatments because her kidneys were still not functioning. Through all of this the family prayed for Cassi's blood pressure to improve on its own so that the vasoconstrictors that were taking such a toll on her extremities could be gradually reduced and eventually discontinued.

Finally, on the fourth day, her blood pressure began to rise, and on the fifth day she came off the vasoconstrictors. This gave the family renewed hope that maybe her fingers and feet would begin to show improvement as she stabilized. In the meantime friends of the family began efforts to rally assistance and support for Cassi. Dan Wylie, Cassi's best friend from high school, set up a trust fund with the help of Cassi's brother-in-law, Britt Cooper. Also, Chris and Rhoda Hauth, Cassi's tae kwon do instructors, began organizing a benefit fund-raiser, one of many fund-raising events organized by the Hauths.

On July 11, the day before Cassi's benefit, she produced urine on her own for the first time, after almost three weeks of daily hemodialysis. While treatments would still be necessary, this was a sign that her kidneys were beginning to function on their own. This was a source of joy for family and friends at the benefit.

The benefit was a huge success. Everyone in attendance agreed that they had never before witnessed such an outpouring of support and compassion. Cars were parked up to half a mile away and people stood in line for up to a half hour just to get in. Between 2,500 and 3,000 people attended, and $22,000 was raised.

At the time of the benefit, Cassi was conscious but still very disoriented and not completely lucid. She had been off the ventilator for about ten days and was able to speak, although at times she hallucinated and was delusional. She was still unaware of her condition. She had not asked about her fingers or toes or about what disease she had. The waiting was very painful for the family. They had no idea how Cassi would respond once she became aware enough to ask. By this time it was certain she would lose a large percentage of all her fingers except for the left thumb. Ironically the left thumb, which was the lone survivor, was the site of the small cut where the bacteria had entered. It was also clear that she would lose her right leg below the knee and one-third of her left foot. Her fingers and toes were completely black and shriveled, with no body heat or pulse. Her right foot, while showing some improvement a few days earlier, had now turned gray. There was a pulse in her heel and on the side of the foot, but a large area on the top of her foot extending up to her shin was without a pulse and cold to the touch.

Finally, on July 13, Cassi asked about her fingers, toes, and foot. When informed that she would most likely lose all of them she responded, "Oh well, I'll just have to deal with it." Her family figured that it would hit her harder later; however, Cassi proved to be far stronger than anyone could have imagined. There were times later that things got to her a bit, but she always pulled out of it, and the way she responded has been an inspiration to all who know her.

On July 14 she was stable enough to move out of ICU. On July 15 she asked her husband and parents what the disease was that she had contracted. When told that she had the flesh-eating bacteria, she burst into tears and praised and thanked God that she was alive.

Cassi had numerous blisterlike sores on her leg that the surgeons were waiting to heal before they amputated the leg in order to provide healthy tissue at the amputation site. The wounds required dressing changes three times a day, and this procedure was painful. Because her right leg was in such considerable pain, she was ready to go ahead with the amputation. Finally the doctors felt that the sores had healed sufficiently to do the surgery.

On July 28 Cassi had surgery to amputate her right leg below the knee and to apply a skin graft taken from her left thigh to the wound on her side. All went well with both procedures. Cassi's sister Stephanie, her son Robbie, Dan, and Cassi's parents were all there the day of the surgery. While she was in recovery, Dan and her parents went in to see her. This was a very emotional time for all of them. Seeing her leg gone for the first time really drove home the terrible tragedy that had happened to her.

For about twenty-four hours after the surgery, there were some problems keeping Cassi's pain under control. She had to wear a sling that kept her left arm immobile for ten days to make sure the graft did not pull lose. This was particularly hard on her because she is very claustrophobic. Recovery went well and after ten days the plastic surgeons removed the bandage from her side. They were pleased to find the graft had taken about 95 percent, which meant further grafting would not be necessary. Also, her leg was healing very well, and there was no sign of infection at either site. Now the only remaining issue was Cassi's fingers and the toes on her left foot. These were being left to resolve themselves, or heal as much as possible before any surgery. They did this to generate the maximum amount of healthy tissue and maximum amount of length on all sites.

Into Rehab

Finally, on August 11, after forty-nine days in the hospital, Cassi was transferred to a rehabilitation center, where she would begin rehab and wait for her last surgery. Cassi's stay at the rehabilitation center consisted of physical therapy, occupational therapy, and mostly waiting. Shortly after arriving at the center, an infection set into her fingers. As a result of this, a very strong course of antibiotics was started to kill the infection and allow more time for regeneration. She required two types of intravenous antibiotics, which had to be given separately, one hour each every eight hours. This made it impossible for Cassi to get any long periods of rest.

The antibiotics did their job, and on August 31, Cassi went to yet another hospital to have her fingers and one third of her foot amputated. It was a four-hour surgery. The surgeon said everything went well and that he was able to remove all of the dead tissue. Cassi was not doing well after the surgery. She was in a lot of pain, and the nurses in recovery were unable to give her enough medication to bring it under control. On top of this, the ambulance company had been called and was standing by to transport her back to the rehabilitation center. It became apparent to the family that this should not have been an outpatient surgery, and Cassi's husband requested she be held overnight so her pain could be properly managed. The anesthesiologist and surgeon recommended she be transported back to the rehabilitation center because they would not be able to stay and take care of her. The nurse gave her one last dose of morphine and sent her on her way.

When Cassi arrived at the rehab center, things went downhill fast. They had only just received her orders for medication. The staff clearly lacked the necessary training or experience to effectively manage a case such as hers. As a result, she experienced much pain that night and the whole family was very upset with the poor manner in which the whole procedure was handled. Finally, a pain management specialist was called in and he was able to help Cassi, so the following days went more smoothly.

Home at Last

On September 9, Cassi was discharged from the rehab center and went home. After being in hospitals for seventy-seven days, she was finally going home to her children, her cat, her dog, and her own bed! There would be no more nurses waking her up in the middle of the night to give her medication. No more doctors waking her up at 5 A.M. to see how she was doing. Needless to say, Dan and Cassi were very happy to be home.

The last months of 1998 were spent trying to get things as close to normal as could be expected. John Batsdorf, of Sierra Orthopedic Lab, put Cassi in a leg with a Flex-Foot, an innovative prosthetic device that allows her to simulate balancing by using a split base so she can rock side to side on her right leg. It also springs at the ankle, allowing her to walk more naturally and giving her more flexibility for going up and down inclines. After she received her first prosthetic leg, she began the process of learning to walk again. This process was slowed considerably due to the fact that not only had she lost her right leg below the knee, she had also lost approximately one-third of her left foot. The left foot became a problem because now she had a much smaller surface to support herself on. The bones that used to be her arch were now being called upon to bear her weight. Also, this made it difficult for her to balance. John came to the rescue and made her an insert for her shoe that would roll the foot into a more natural position. This helped considerably, and further improvements have enabled Cassi to begin walking more naturally. She still walks with a limp, because her foot could take up to a year to completely heal, but she has already made considerable progress.

Cassi found she could still play her keyboard despite losing 90 percent of all of her fingers. John Batsdorf helped her further with this by designing some extensions on the fingers necessary for her to reach all of the notes. She found that she really could do all of the things she did before. Every time something came up that she couldn't do, a way was found for her to do it. She was driving in no time, and her father helped by modifying a device that moved the gas pedal to the left side of the floorboard so she could use her good foot to operate it. He also modified a curling iron and constantly came up with gadgets and ideas to help make things easier for her.

On New Year's Eve 1998, the whole family went out for the night to celebrate. All holidays have extra special meaning for Cassi's family now. Nothing will ever be taken for granted again. It was a special night. Her family celebrated not only the new year but also the special life that God had spared. They also celebrated the newfound love and closeness they each felt for one another. Cassi danced for the first time and looked very beautiful. It was a very special night, indeed.

Victory

Cassi continued to improve through 1999. Her walking has slowly but surely improved, and her endurance and pain continue to improve also. On March 9, 1999, Cassi returned to work. This was a big step in her recovery and brought her enormous satisfaction. Cassi's leg will continue to lose the buildup of fluid, but this may take up to a year. Because of this her prosthetic leg has a temporary socket that will allow her residual leg to shrink. In time, her leg will stabilize, and she will be fitted for a prosthesis with a permanent socket.

Cassi hopes to return to tae kwon do this summer. Special gloves will be made to protect her hands while punching. Moves and techniques will be modified some to allow for the lack of fingers and flexibility on her feet.

Cassi's incredible vitality and positive attitude are examples of the human spirit that often emerges during the ordeal of necrotizing fasciitis. While Cassi's recovery may seem incredible and unlikely, it's actually typical. It's only the magnitude of her lasting effects of the NF that makes her story different from many others. We have encountered hundreds of NF victims who echo the statement, "I'm so thankful to be alive." Then the healing begins.

There is no such thing as a "mild case" of NF. Those who are stricken have been through a harrowing experience of pain and healing made even worse by the social stigma of having to explain "necrotizing fasciitis" after it is all over.

Cassi is an exemplary portrait of survival. We have told her story to many people who need to know that "everything can be OK" after NF. Looking at her, no one can disagree.

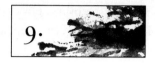

9.

Continuing the Recovery Process after Hospitalization

LAST JULY, I was diagnosed with necrotizing fasciitis-myositis. I was in the hospital for three weeks, two of which I spent in the intensive care unit. It was the most traumatic experience of my lifetime. I know I am one of the lucky ones to have made it out of this with no muscle loss or amputation. I do have incision lines from the debridement, lining the inner and outer parts of both legs. When I left the hospital, I was using a walker, and I still had excruciating pain in my hip. Today, I am racing around after my infant and toddler. I wish I could say I am 100 percent better, but I still have a lot of things to work through. I still have mental and physical scars that I am trying to recover from.

—Kelly

You're finally discharged from the hospital—blinking in the daylight, breathing in the fresh air, taking in the world you knew before you were stricken. What a welcome change from the sights, smells, and sounds of the hospital! Although you are probably still quite weak and in pain and you tire easily, you are still overjoyed at having beaten this potentially life-threatening disease. But the battle is far from over. Recovery from the effects of the infection takes some time as well.

There are so many levels of recovery: physical, emotional, spiritual, and social. Each level of recovery takes time and attention. In this chapter we will focus on the physical aspects. The recovery process will vary from person to person, but in general, the process is four-pronged. It consists of getting the body back to optimum health, coping with complications and residual effects of the infection, and undergoing reconstructive surgery and fitting for prosthetic devices. We'll discuss each of these aspects of physical recovery in this chapter and offer unique insight from NF survivors as well.

Getting Back to Optimum Health after NF

After surviving a battle with NF, one's immune system, mind, and body are severely exhausted. There may be damage to one's heart, lungs, kidneys, or other internal organs that require special attention. As a survivor, you may feel like a fleet of trucks hit you—and you have the scars to prove it. In order to return to a normal life, it is important that you concentrate on getting your body and mind back to optimum health.

The Rehabilitation Center

NF patients who are considered out of danger, but who still require 24-hour close medical monitoring, IV medication, and frequent dressing changes, may be transferred to an aftercare facility such as a skilled nursing-care or rehabilitation center. The length of stay will vary according to patient needs, but could be a period of several days or even weeks. One of the most important goals of the rehabilitation center staff, in addition to physical healing, is to encourage self-motivation and independence in the home in day-to-day tasks. Most rehabilitation centers are fully staffed to provide for the unique needs of post-NF patients, including physical, nutritional, and often psychological therapy.

Besides the medical and physical needs of recuperating patients, there are any number of tasks that an NF patient is unlikely to be able to do alone, such as washing his or her hair or just getting dressed. The rehabilitation center is also useful in helping a person with these tasks until he or she is able to be self-sufficient. These centers are a blessing for many people, and let them bridge the gap between release from the hospital and wellness.

Home-Care Nursing

When an NF patient is well enough to go home but is still in need of skilled medical treatment such as wound dressing changes or intravenous administration of antibiotics, home-care nursing may be ordered. Depending upon the extent of the injuries, home care may also include housekeeping and personal assistance in day-to-day activities. It may even include physical therapy.

The family of the NF victim can be a tremendous help to the home health care staff. Family members can share their observations regarding the patient's day-to-day progress, including the patient's eating and sleeping habits, pain, psychological adjustment, and other factors relating to physical healing.

If an NF patient lives alone, and health insurance permits, home-care nursing may continue for quite some time. Those survivors with live-in or nearby family members, however, are often entrusted with wound care after a period of time, with occasional visits by a home-care aide perhaps.

Nutrition to Promote Healing

During treatment, NF patients are often fed through a feeding tube, resulting in weight loss and the lack of essential nutrients that are necessary for normal daily activities, not to mention healing. In order to get our bodies back to optimum condition during the long physical and emotional recovery process, it is extremely important that we pay close attention to our nutritional needs. Nutritional healing does not have to be an expensive or complicated process, as you'll read, but because each person is different, it is important to consult a qualified physician or nutritionist to discuss an appropriate dietary plan before starting. There are some nutrition basics that we all should adhere to, however.

Sufficient protein intake is paramount for the recovery process. We spoke with Alan Cohen, M.D., an expert in nutrition and holistic medicine practicing in Milford, Connecticut, regarding the specific needs of patients recovering from NF. "Protein is severely depleted when fighting a severe illness," he said. "Therefore, to strengthen and heal the body, it is important to increase protein intake during physical recovery." Sources of protein include red meat, fish, chicken, eggs, milk, and soy products (such as tofu and tempeh). Combining these foods with other sources of protein, such as brown rice, raw seeds, beans, lentils, peas, and whole grains, can satisfy protein requirements. Protein shakes—from the fashionable and expensive to old-fashioned standbys such as Carnation Instant Breakfast drinks—also are abundant on the market lately.

Coldwater fish (like salmon, cod, sardines, and mackerel) are preferred as protein sources over shellfish because of their high concentration of omega-3 fatty acids, which promote healing and bolster the immune system. Table 7.1 below lists some common foods and their protein content. A person's body weight and level of activity affect the amount of protein needed on a daily basis, which is between 60 and 100 grams. Less active people require less protein.

TABLE 7.1. THE PROTEIN CONTENT OF SELECTED FOODS	
Food	Protein Content
Halibut, 3 oz	22.7 g
Salmon, 3 oz	21.6 g
Ground beef, lean, 3 oz	21.2 g
Shrimp, 3 oz	17.3 g
Ham, lean, 3 oz	15.9 g
Kidney beans, 1 cup	15.4 g
Black beans, 1 cup	15.4 g
Cottage cheese, 1/2 cup	14.0 g
Yogurt, low-fat, 1 cup	11.9 g
Tofu, 1/2 cup	11.0 g
Milk, all types, 1 cup	8.0 g
Egg, medium	6.0 g

Certain vitamins and other supplements are also recommended to fortify the body during physical recovery. Vitamin A is a fat-soluble vitamin involved in the formation and maintenance of healthy skin, hair, and mucous membranes. It will also aid in maintaining healthy bones and teeth. Sources of vitamin A are dark-green vegetables and deep-yellow fruits, grain products, and milk and milk products.

Vitamin C is very important to wound healing as well as the formation of collagen found in the skin, ligaments, cartilage, vertebral discs, joint linings, capillary walls, bones, and teeth. Vitamin C also helps maintain healthy blood vessels. Vitamin C is easily destroyed during cooking, especially with water. Lightly steam or sauté your produce in order to retain most of the vitamin C content. To retain the full vitamin C content of foods, it is best to eat them raw. The best sources of vitamin C include broccoli, Brussels sprouts, collard greens, kale, turnip greens, sweet potatoes, and citrus fruits. The fruits with the highest natural concentrations are citrus fruits, rose hips, and acerola cherries, followed by papayas, cantaloupes, and strawberries.

Vitamin E has a long list of benefits for patients recovering after NF, including the stimulation of the immune system, wound healing, and protection against secondary infections. It also maintains the integrity of vitamin A in the body and promotes normal clotting of blood. It is important to note, however, that vitamin E levels are dependent upon proper amounts of zinc in the body. Excellent sources of vitamin E include almonds, apricot oil, corn oil, cottonseed oil, hazelnuts, margarine, peanut oil, safflower nuts, sunflower seeds, walnuts, wheat germ, and whole-wheat flour.

Zinc is also important to wound healing. In the initial stages of healing, 40 milligrams of the mineral twice a day is the recommended dosage. After four to six weeks the dosage is cut to only 40 milligrams per day. Because copper and zinc work together, it is also important to increase copper 2 to 3 milligrams per day while taking extra zinc.

The supplement coenzyme Q_{10} is also beneficial for survivors of NF. This highly acclaimed supplement increases the oxygen supply to the tissues, stimulates the immune system, and aids in wound healing. The dosage recommended is 50 milligrams per day.

Our bodies typically work in harmony with friendly bacteria in our intestinal tract that aid digestion and help to keep the body healthy. Because antibiotics wipe out these good bacteria, they must be replaced in supplement form. *Lactobacillus acidophilus* and *Lactobacillus bifidus* are two beneficial supplemental forms of bacteria. It is important that the product label state that "live cultures" or "viable cultures" are present. The recommended dosage is two capsules, twice per day.

Another important supplement that Dr. Cohen recommends for those recovering from NF is omega-3 essential fatty acids (EFAs). Omega-3 EFAs, as mentioned earlier, are known to promote healing and strengthen the immune system. Flaxseed oil, either in tablet or liquid form, is an excellent source of omega-3 EFAs. Keep in mind that one tablespoon of liquid flaxseed oil is the equivalent of approximately eight tablets.

A final suggestion that Dr. Cohen offers to NF survivors to ensure that the body is functioning at the best possible level is to increase fiber and water intake. "The amount of fiber that is comfortable for people can vary dramatically," warns Dr. Cohen. "Stomach pain and cramping should signal too much fiber, so you should reduce the amount by increments of ten grams or so. The average amount is about 30 grams per day." Increasing your water intake is equally important. Drinking eight glasses of water per day every single day can do wonders for rejuvenating the body.

Wound Care

The care of wounds caused by debridement surgery and amputation is a significant part of the physical recovery of NF. Changing wound dressings is unpleasant to say the least, but it must be performed carefully and attentively to avoid secondary infections and to promote healing of the wounds.

Ideally an NF patient would have a home-care aide to attend to his or her wounds and change the dressings; however, that can not always be the case. Quite often the patient's family must be in charge of wound care. Don't fret. As long as some general guidelines are followed, laypeople can safely and effectively tend to an NF patient's wounds. Set aside a private, peaceful, and clean area of the house to change dressings. Keep all materials (disposable sterile tweezers, sterile gloves, saline, gauze, etc.) in a readily accessible and clean "toolbox" that is off-limits to curious children. Wear a mask if you are showing any signs of sickness, including a cold.

The general rules for caring for an amputation wound are to keep the site clean, moist, and covered to protect it from injury. "Many people are under the mistaken assumption that wounds should be left open to the air to heal," explains Tamara Fishman, M.D., of North Miami Beach, Florida, a podiatric wound-care consultant and director of the Wound Care Institute, a nonprofit organization for all facets of wound care. "But wounds heal faster and with less potential for infection in a moist environment."

Although your home may be clean, it is next to impossible to obtain a completely sterile environment for changing dressings. Therefore it is extremely important to exercise the highest level of caution to ensure that conditions are as clean as possible for changing wound dressings in the home. For example, if you are changing the patient's dressings in his or her bed, it is important to wash the bedclothes before the next dressing change. Furthermore, the patient must be careful not to sleep or otherwise remain in dressings that have excessive wound drainage, even if it means replacing the dressings three or more times per day. Of course, hand-washing—before and after wound care—is of paramount importance as well.

In most circumstances you must first cleanse or flush the wound with plain saline solution before putting new dressings on it. Some physicians recommend treating the wound next with such antiseptic solutions as peroxide, Dakin's solution, or Betadine, while other wound care specialists feel these products can be more hurtful than helpful. "It is believed that these solutions disrupt the normal healing process by interfering with the formation of fibroblasts, the cells that produce connective tissues," explains Dr. Fishman. "I do not recommend their use for long-term wound care—at the most, five to seven days."

The amputated area should then be carefully inspected for any changes that could signal a problem. Is there increased drainage? If so, is there a foul odor? Is there any change to the overall condition of the wound? Is there increased pain? Changes must be immediately brought to the attention of the treating physician for further analysis, particularly if the patient reports increased pain, increased drainage, swelling, and/or fever.

To keep the area moist, a hydrogel (a thick water-based gel) should be applied to the wound with a freshly gloved hand. Sterile gauze should then be wrapped snugly, but not tightly, around the wound. Paper tape for binding the gauze to the skin is a better choice than other types of medical tape, as it is less irritating to the skin. A covering such as a stocking, stockinette, or Spandage (a highly elastic, non-latex tubular bandage that does not require tape), pulled over or wrapped around the limb to protect it from potential injury, is typically the last step.

Dr. Fishman explains that used dressings should be treated as contaminated waste: Put them into a separate plastic bag, and discard immediately. And *never, ever reuse dressing material, even if it appears to be perfectly clean.* For some patients on a very limited budget with little insurance reimbursement for materials, this may be a temptation.

You can expect to have to continue changing your dressings for up to three months or more. During this time, bathing should be limited. "Wound-care specialists have varying opinions, however, I tell my patients absolutely no baths until the wound is healed. I even prefer no showers either, as shampoos and soaps can cause irritation to the open wound," explains Dr. Fishman. "For the first month at least, I recommend sponge baths only for my wound care patients."

Dr. Fishman offers some final advice to NF survivors who are responsible for their own wound care. "Keep in mind that you, the patient, are equally responsible for healing as the doctor. By managing wound care carefully, keeping track of symptoms, reporting problems, and expressing concerns to your physician, you are fulfilling a very important role in your own health care. Remember also that you have been through a lot physically and mentally, and are not superhuman. Create a safe, trauma-free environment in order to let your wounds heal."

Deep wounds require special treatment, as they take longer to heal. Wound care in this circumstance is known as "packing." Essentially, the wound is left open and allowed to heal from the inside out. A product such as ribbon gauze, which resembles a tangle of shoelaces, is used to "pack" the wound, as we'll describe in the next paragraph.

Deep wounds should be cared for in a manner similar to amputation wounds. After cleaning a wound, examine its condition—with the assistance of a flashlight if necessary. Any changes in the wound should be documented and immediately reported to the patient's physician. If such symptoms exist, then the wound should not be repacked until the patient sees his or her physician. If everything appears normal, however, the wound should be repacked and carefully covered until the next dressing change.

With both amputation sites and deep wounds, if dressing changes are painful, it is sometimes recommended that the patient take pain medication about an hour or so prior to the scheduled time for the next dressing change. In the beginning, dressings may need to be changed twice a day or more, and then the need will taper off as the wound heals.

Care of Skin Grafts

Skin grafts are generally cared for by the plastic surgeon or his or her staff in the early stages. Skin grafts are fragile, prone to infections, and must be carefully monitored. It can sometimes take several weeks before it is determined that a skin graft is going to "take," and improper dressing changes can affect the success rate. The dressings must be changed rather infrequently. Eventually, however, once the graft is determined to be successful, dressing changes are handled at home by the patient or his or her family in much the same as other sterile dressing changes.

Donor Site Wounds

Donor site wounds are the "tire-track–like" scars that are left at the location from which the skin has been harvested for a skin graft. The area where the skin is taken is generally covered with a material such as polymer film—thin, elastic, adhesive sheets of polyurethane. These transparent sheets are semipermeable, protecting the wound from bacteria and allowing the wound to "breathe" while keeping it moist, which is beneficial to healing. As time goes on, the use of polymer film is discontinued, and the wound is cared for with the above standard procedures. Healing is slow, uncomfortable, and sometimes troublesome. First of all, if the donor site is located on the thighs or buttocks, it is very difficult to let the wound heal unhindered by clothing. Moreover, large bandages do not stay in areas like the buttocks or thighs with ease. While some NF patients' donor sites heal with no problem, others say that the donor site wounds are the most painful part of healing.

Silvadene, or silver sulfadiazine, is an effective prescription antimicrobial cream used to protect against a wide range of bacteria, yeast, and fungi. Physicians may prescribe this topical medication, or a similar one such as bacitracin, Bactroban, or Neosporin to promote wound healing and to stave off secondary infections.

Physical and Occupational Therapy

My NF experience began three years ago as a slip and fall causing massive bruising in my left lower leg. The course of my illness was slow and rocky. I kept my leg and my life, but have some loss of muscle and lymphatic system in the affected area. The best decision I made during my recovery was to insist upon physical therapy. Not only did it build strength, but my therapist also broke down scar tissue that had formed in the area. It took me a full two years to recover.

—Cindy

Physical therapists, who in the past have generally dealt with lower-body mobility, and occupational therapists, who in the past have been concerned with task performance and general upper mobility including that of hands, arms, and shoulders, are an integral part of the recovery process for NF victims.

We say "in the past" because, although these guidelines are generally true, today one finds that the lines have become less definite and that therapy is more of a team effort. For this reason we will simply refer to these health care providers as "therapists." Their jobs must be very rewarding, as they guide patients toward adjusting to, accepting, and eventually overcoming their new physical challenges—including learning to walk again. A strong foundation of mutual respect, teamwork, trust, and patience between the therapist and patient is critical throughout the long and sometimes tedious procedures that are the heart of physical therapy. Together, the therapist and patient perform hours of repetitive exercise to encourage tiny degrees of improvement after weeks of bending, stretching, range of motion exercises, desensitizing of wounds, taping, and massage.

Each of these functions can play into the final result of a patient's recovery of normal function. These important factors can make the difference in whether a person can bend at the knee, make a fist, or otherwise regain normal movement.

To understand the role of physical and occupational therapy for NF patients, we spoke to Lana Keiser, OTR, CHT (Registered Occupational Therapist and Certified Hand Therapist) and Shelly Davis, OTR, of Novacare in Grand Rapids, Michigan. Shelly was the therapist that treated co-author Donna Batdorff, and Lana has treated five cases of NF.

Lana stressed that it is never too early for a therapist to be involved in a patient's care. "We should be there from day one," Lana explained. "We can help from the very beginning with decisions on splinting, dressing changes, and exercise that the patient can tolerate." While it depends on the facility, many doctors prefer the therapist to be involved from the very beginning to assist with wound care.

"The therapist is right there in the whirlpool with a patient," Lana explained. "It's also important to get a patient's joints moving as soon as possible. There is no reason not to move a wound; you need to move the joints to keep a person as loose as possible and to help prevent scar contractures."

The only time that a patient should not be moving is after grafting, according to Shelly. At that time the therapist is often present in the operating room helping to create the splint that will immobilize the grafted area of the patient's body. A graft generally needs to be left alone for three to five days, after which the therapy can resume. The therapist even takes part in debriding the wounds, changing dressings, ongoing wound management, exercises, and patient-needs assessment.

Scar-tissue formation is a major concern for NF survivors. There are two major scar complications that occur: adhesion and contracture. Adhesion refers to a situation in which a thickening of tissue occurs and the collagen fibers adhere to the tissue below the scar. A contracture is a scar that tightens up or shortens because it has not been exercised and stretched. Working with a physical therapist early on after wound healing is extremely beneficial, because the longer one waits to begin therapy, the harder it can be to reverse the tightening of joints and abnormal formation of scar tissue. Scars are generally considered mature and not respondent to therapy after about six months. It is important to try to manipulate scars early in the process prior to that time. There are many things that a skilled therapist can do to help keep a scar from binding, which would inhibit motion later on. These methods can begin in the hospital, according to Lana. "There's no reason that compression (which is important in scar management) cannot be done over bandages." For example, keeping a scar supple by massage and the application of soft, gel-like silicone sheets (such as Elastimar) is helpful in scar management. Elastimar is a "Silly Putty–like" material that can be pressed on a scarred area and will conform exactly to its contours. It then hardens, and is taped onto the area to create compression.

Coban (a special tape used in therapy) is also helpful in scar compression, which helps scar tissue form a neater, more uniform scar.

Lana explains that scar tissue is so difficult to manage because normal skin is constructed in rows and columns, while scar tissue forms in a haphazard way which tends to cause uneven skin texture. "There is a window of opportunity in scar management that needs to be respected," Lana explained. "A scar continues to change and mature for twelve to eighteen months, and the management of that scar needs to be maintained the entire time." Sometimes a lot of progress can be seen and things are going smoothly when suddenly a scar can thicken. "This is why constant monitoring is necessary," Lana says. Massage of scar tissue can also be helpful in training the fibers of a scar to "lie down" and form more in the pattern of healthy tissue. The lighter the skin, the smoother the scarring is likely to be. Lana noted that people with dark skin, particularly African-Americans, tend to have more trouble with scarring.

It's also important to keep scars out of the sun. If a scar gets red, it will take on a burnlike appearance and it will not fade. This is true for a full eighteen months after injury.

A compression garment may also be necessary to reduce the swelling that is often part of the post-NF experience. It may take months of compression, massage, and natural elimination for swelling to subside. There are special commercially produced compression garments that are custom-made to fit a patient. The therapist determines when the timing is right for such a garment, and fits the patient for it. While swelling is often an issue, it generally subsides unless the lymph system has been affected, resulting in chronic lymphedema—a topic we discuss later in this chapter.

Another role of the therapist is to help with restoring the sense of touch to the newly scarred tissue. Desensitizing wounds is one of the ways that therapists help a patient regain normal function. The damaged tissue of an NF victim is, of course, very tender. Even the pressure of a pant leg's fabric, or resting a hand on a sofa cushion, may be too painful in the beginning. In an effort to reorient damaged tissue with the sense of touch, the therapist will introduce a number of exercises, such as asking the patient to stroke a small piece of foam rubber, or dragging cotton balls over the sensitive area and gradually increasing pressure as the patient adjusts to the sensation. When the foam rubber or cotton is tolerable, the patient may graduate to a pencil eraser and touch it lightly over the area, and then increase pressure as tolerance improves. Other exercises may include rolling an empty roll-on deodorant bottle over the skin, or touching various fabrics, beginning with soft ones like cotton or silk and graduating to harsher textures like canvas or burlap.

Moving the limb through light moveable objects, like a bowl of dry lentils, rice, coins, or buttons can also help and build up tolerance. A machine is also used that exposes skin to heated cornhusks that move at a frenzied pace in an enclosed container. This method, called fluidotherapy, is also used to heat tissue so as to make stretching and bending easier in range-of-motion exercises.

In some cases hypersensitivity is not an issue, but rather loss of sensitivity has occurred. "You cannot regain feeling if the nerves are no longer there," Shelly explained. "In that case our role reverts to education. We need to remind people of the hazards that can occur due to the lack of sensitivity." For instance, such patients must be taught not to test water with a finger that is not sensitive, and to be careful while smoking.

The importance of stretching and bending of a patient's scarred areas cannot be stressed enough. Exercise and movement are the keys to restoring normal function. This may include bending of the joints, use of splints to hold joints in certain positions, or use of tape to hold a body part in a stretched position for a period of seconds, which later graduates to minutes as range increases. Therapists also perform manipulation to simulate range of motion, for instance by picking up a leg or arm and moving it in circles out from its rotation point.

This is the most challenging part of therapy for both the patient and the therapist because there is generally some discomfort involved. "Inflicting pain is definitely the most challenging part of our work," Lana said. She explained that the therapist walks a fine line. "You want to stretch or push a person enough to do some good, but you can't go too far or they won't come back."

Therapists are also there to assist the NF patient in adjusting to life as an amputee. This might include retraining the remaining arm, hand, or fingers to perform simple tasks, such as holding a fork, writing, and buttoning clothes. It might also involve teaching patients new ways to do old tasks as simple as opening a carton of milk and as complex as walking. The therapist also plays a role in determining when a prosthetic device would be useful, what type of device would be best, how to use the device, and determining when the timing is right to measure the area of the body for the prosthetic device.

A therapist's work with amputees might also involve helping a patient walk with a prosthetic leg, or adjusting to using a prosthetic arm. Getting used to prosthetic devices can be frustrating and physically painful. Again, the relationship forged between the physical therapist and the patient is invaluable.

The length of time that an NF patient should remain in therapy depends greatly on need, but unfortunately it is often dictated by an insurance company. Some insurance companies will only pay for two months of therapy. This puts the NF patient at a clear disadvantage, as more time is almost always needed. If insurance were not a factor, generally speaking, a person should stay in therapy as long as he or she continues to show improvement.

Success in therapy depends on several factors, not the least of which is a positive attitude. "I think a positive attitude is one of the most important things," Shelly says. "If a person does not have a good attitude, it makes everything harder. We try to bring people out of negativity by always emphasizing the positive aspects." Family members' cooperation, involvement, and support are also important, as these individuals can help with wound care and exercises in the home.

"There is so much (therapists) do in helping the NF patient," Lana said. "Our role is from start to finish. From day one, when they are stricken with the infection, until they go home independent in life, dressing, eating, and working. We are involved from start to finish with the goal of getting that patient to the best physical level they can be and in the best day-to-day living situation they can achieve. We are counselors, educators, facilitators, and motivators."

Hand Therapy

A significant amount of NF occurs in the hands and arms, and the job of the Certified Hand Therapist bears mentioning. Particularly if the hand and fingers are affected, a Certified Hand Therapist should be the therapist of choice. The hand is the only part of the body that has a special certification for therapists.

As hand surgeons became more and more skilled and began doing more and more involved procedures, they began to want specialized therapists to help get the end results they hoped for with their surgeries. The first hand therapy certification testing was done in 1992 by the American Society of Hand Therapists. Before one can even sit for the certification test, one needs to have an occupational therapy certification, and to have been practicing for more than five years, and in that time to have worked with hands for at least 2,000 hours. It's difficult: many people study for a long time and still do not pass the test.

For NF patients recuperating with hand injuries, to work with a certified hand therapist is a wise decision. Lana puts it into perspective, "A tiny scar on the foot probably won't get in the way of much, but a tiny scar on the hand can affect whether or not you can grab a bottle of milk out of the refrigerator."

Reconstructive Surgery

A year or more after the physical wounds have healed, an NF patient may opt for reconstructive surgery to improve the appearance of his or her skin or to correct residual problems such as adhesions, scar contracture, or discomfort associated with an amputated limb, such as bone spurs. Reconstructive surgery is performed by a plastic surgeon and in many cases is conducted as outpatient surgery.

Reconstructive and scar-revision surgery, which attempt to minimize the appearance of scars, can certainly reduce the appearance of many scars caused by a traumatic illness such as NF; however, in patients with substantial amounts of scarring, skin grafting, and residual donor site scars, the procedure may be only mildly beneficial. It is important for NF patients to be realistic about the outcome. Unfortunately, because scar revision surgery may be interpreted as a cosmetic procedure, it may not be covered by many insurance plans, so make sure you speak with your insurance company beforehand.

Prosthetics

Deciding whether or not to use prosthetic devices after limb or digit loss is a personal choice. For many, the trauma of physical loss can be lessened by restoring the natural appearance of still having the missing limb. Many others find that they can learn to function well without an artificial limb, and still others use their prosthesis only occasionally.

Many companies produce limbs, hooks, hands, and feet that are functional, if far from looking realistic or feeling comfortable. However, there are companies emerging in the marketplace that utilize modern technology and artistry to create beautiful lifelike fingers, hands, feet, legs, etc. We present few actual recommendations in this book; however, we feel compelled to mention a company in Brandon, MS, as a resource for these amazing, hard-to-find prosthetic devices. The company, Alatheia Prosthetic Rehabilitation Center, specializes in 100-percent lifelike prostheses that can cover scarring on a limb, be fitted with functional devices, or be worn alone. Coauthor Donna Batdorff has prosthetic fingers that cannot be detected, even when people are challenged to guess which fingers are not "real." Information regarding Alatheia Prosthetic Rehabilitation Center is provided in the Resources section of this book.

The process of being fitted with a prosthetic limb is multifaceted. Carol Wallace, author of *Challenged by Amputation: Embracing a New Life,* offers the following information in her book:

- Communicate with your prosthetist. In all likelihood, you will be spending three to six months working out the problems of your first prosthetic limb with him or her and visiting at least once a year thereafter for prosthetic maintenance and adjustment. Failure to maintain a proper limb-and-socket fit can result in many physical problems, including skin breakdown and ulceration.
- Describe both the life you led and the plans you have mapped out for the future. If you're active, you will need a strong limb, one that will hold up while participating in sports, heavy work, or other activities. If you're less active, you may want a lightweight or cosmetic limb. Cosmetic limbs usually match your skin color and are sculpted to match your other leg. Heavy-duty legs are usually made of hard plastic with hydraulic workings. Some people request two replacement limbs, one for use in sports, such as skiing or running, and a lighter one for everyday activities. Other limbs, such as peg legs or shower legs (prosthetics with no moving parts, designed for convenience), while not cosmetically correct, are good for balancing in the shower and getting around the house.
- Additional issues of particular concern to women include choosing a heel height for all of your shoes to maximize balance, selecting the

shaping of the limb, and determining possible solutions to the problem of color differences between the prosthesis and your skin tone, such as double-thickness pantyhose and textured tights. Your menstrual cycle may also cause your residual limb to swell, which will affect the fit of your limb. With an above-the-knee prosthesis, sanitary pads may be difficult to wear because the leg fits so tightly against the groin.

• Some insurance companies don't cover prostheses; others pay for only one in a lifetime. The Veterans Administration provides only a limited number of limbs. Medicare also has limits. Since it's crucial that you get what you need, you must speak up and be willing to wrangle with your insurance provider, if necessary, to be heard loud and clear. A good-fitting prosthesis can be the difference between being totally incapacitated and totally functioning. Some people (especially kids) can go through a prosthesis a year. Others have several ineffective prostheses made before they find someone who can make the right one. With revisions to the socket every year or so, sometimes a prosthesis can last several years. Lifestyle also dictates the usage and type of devices. For example, athletic people often have two or three legs for different activities. Others have cosmetic legs that look like a real leg, but aren't made for rough activities.

For those fortunate enough to survive NF without long-term organ damage or amputation, getting back to a normal life—work, children, friends, hobbies, sports—is just a matter of allowing enough time for wounds to heal and stamina to return to acceptable levels. Residual skin damage and scarring may interfere with some activities, perhaps restricting lifting or vigorous exercise. Other survivors who have lost limbs and/or suffer from permanent organ damage may find that they must adapt to drastic changes to their lifestyles, careers, relationships, and activity levels. There are many resources available to NF survivors regarding amputation, reconstructive surgery, prosthetics, nutrition, filing for disability coverage, etc., that can offer guidance and advice for the patient through the physical aspects of surviving necrotizing fasciitis. We encourage survivors to investigate as much as possible to find what works for them.

Any survivor of NF will tell you that the physical aspect of recovery is just a fraction of what one must go through. In the next chapter we will discuss the issues of emotional, psychological, and spiritual recovery for both the NF survivor and the family of those who have lost the battle to the disease.

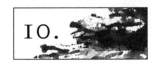

Psychological, Emotional, and Spiritual Recovery

⑥

Ways of coping with the psychological, emotional, and spiritual impact of surviving necrotizing fasciitis are as diverse as the NF victims themselves. Some people wake up in the intensive care unit with missing limbs and simply thank God that they are alive. Others may suffer a wide spectrum of emotions, such as anger, profound depression, and self-pity. One fact is clear, however: No matter how the NF victim ultimately deals with the experience, he or she is forever changed. This change is not only physical. Frequently, NF survivors undergo a spiritual transformation, finding themselves becoming more in touch with God and their inner spirituality.

Throughout this chapter we try to provide guideposts for NF survivors and their loved ones to assist them along the path toward psychological, emotional, and spiritual recovery after NF. We call upon the advice of experts in the fields of trauma recovery, psychotherapy, and spirituality for their unique insight. NF survivors and the loved ones of those who have died also share their personal stories and suggestions.

Psychological and Emotional Recovery

Looking in the mirror for the first time after surviving NF can be a painful experience rife with raw and unexpected emotions. Throughout hospitalization, NF patients are often detached from their feelings. They are surrounded by a flock of nurses and doctors with their senses dulled by painkillers and sedatives, and are often unconscious. As they are slowly guided out of danger, many—despite their physical pain, fear, and loneliness—are determined to put on a brave face for their loved ones who hover over their hospital beds, worried and frightened about losing them. However, their detached state can quickly dissolve into a rush of overwhelming emotions when they are finally released from the hospital and come to realize how their lives have been changed. They may discover that they can no longer walk, dance, play sports, drive a car, work, make love, or enjoy many of the pleasures in life that they may have taken for granted before they were stricken.

Perhaps you may have discovered that, despite your desire for privacy, you are making headline news. Local newspapers and television and radio stations keep the phone ringing off the hook to talk to the amazing survivor of the flesh-eating bacteria. Neighbors may stare and, in their fear and lack of understanding about the disease, avoid you like you were a leper of biblical times. Your loved ones may try their hardest to be loving and supportive, but despite the very best of intentions, comforting words and heartfelt advice cannot allay the inner turmoil you are experiencing.

Your psychological, emotional, and spiritual health is of paramount importance to your ultimate recovery. You cannot ignore, deny, gloss over, laugh away, or shrug off the need to grieve for what you have lost in your life. You have suffered a truly traumatic event—with life-changing effects—and you must give yourself permission to feel the emotions of your loss, and must learn to cope with the tremendous changes going on in your life.

But what can you expect to feel after such a devastating experience as necrotizing fasciitis? For many NF survivors, recuperating after NF can be a tumultuous roller-coaster ride of mixed emotions, creating wild dips and turns in how we feel from day to day, or even hour to hour. For instance, deep down, a survivor may be grateful to be alive but may also feel angry or saddened that he or she can no longer walk without a prosthesis. In the following pages we will explore some feelings that NF survivors commonly experience.

Anger and Frustration

I was angry for a long time after my experience with necrotizing fasciitis. I managed to resolve much of that anger by writing a letter to the insurance company, which automatically resulted in an internal audit of my case.

—Cyndy

The intensity of feelings of anger and frustration that NF survivors experience can be quite dramatic and difficult to deal with. Survivors may be angry that their once healthy and attractive bodies are forever marred by shark-bite–like scarring and/or missing fingers or limbs. Perhaps the anger may be due to the fact that their independence is replaced with reliance on others for help in routine tasks such as bathing and dressing. Or sometimes people cannot give a name to the reason for their frustration, but they know it's there.

Suppressed anger can manifest as anxiety and/or depression. One may not realize that in actuality he or she is angry about their losses. Feelings of anger following a traumatic loss are normal. As we'll discuss later, the absence of anger, including a "too-positive" attitude or the lack of emotions all together, can delay the psychological and emotional healing process.

Talking honestly and openly about your feelings with a trusted loved one or therapist may help you cope with your emotions. While it will take time for the feelings of anger and frustration to pass, the old adage "A problem shared is a problem halved" holds true. Talking helps to unknot your emotions and can give you a new perspective on your experience and your future.

Many people also find that keeping a journal is quite therapeutic in coping with anger as well as other emotions. Be sure to write freely and honestly. Allow yourself to be angry and the words will tumble out, and eventually so will the negative feelings.

Depression and Sadness

My scar is 23 inches long, 13 inches wide, and 2 inches deep down the right side of my body. The top of my right leg is numb, as is my back and half of my abdomen. Three fingers on my right hand are numb because of nerve damage. I feel I could go on forever telling you what happened. I try to keep a brave face for everyone else. I would often go to bed at night and cry myself to sleep—that is, if I could sleep. I was on sleeping tablets for a long time. I felt like everyone was sick of listening to me, even though no one said so. I would cry for no reason and I think that was hard for everyone to understand.

—Lee

Depression and sadness are debilitating emotions that not only leave us living at only a fraction of our true potential but can also have repercussions on our physical healing. Episodes of depression can be either mild (feeling blue) or severe (thoughts of suicide), or anywhere in between. All of us feel blue now and then in reaction to certain life events, but quickly rebound to our "old selves" again. However, when feelings of sadness, worthlessness, guilt, helplessness, and hopelessness become chronic (lasting longer than a few days), it is important that we seek help.

Feelings of depression can be exacerbated by nutritional deficiencies. The prolonged use of medications can also drain the body of energy, resulting in feelings of mental fatigue, difficulty concentrating, and depression. Ensuring that our bodies are in the best possible condition, as discussed in Chapter 9, can do wonders for our mental health as well.

The treatment options available for people suffering from depression are wide and varied, ranging from traditional psychotherapy and antidepressant drug therapy to alternative methods like Emotional Freedom Techniques (EFT). We will discuss some of these options later on in this chapter.

One survivor, Bob, from California, struggled with depression for months after his bout with NF. He gained weight, was constantly fatigued, and had a dim outlook on life. Then Bob was invited to work out with a friend at a local gym. While at first he was reluctant to show his rather dramatic-looking scars in public, after a while they no longer seemed important. In time he made friends with whom he shared his experience with the flesh-eating bacteria. Bob dedicated himself to an exercise program and found his spirits lifting more and more each day. Exercise had an added benefit: He lost over 60 pounds and has an energy level he never dreamed of attaining before.

Many people have reported to us that reaching out to other survivors was extremely therapeutic and helped them in overcoming their depression. Our Web site, www.nnff.org, has brought together a great number of NF survivors throughout the world, as well as the loved ones of those who died. Through e-mail and our Web site's chat room, people affected by NF find support, comfort, and kinship. We have seen the bond between survivors of NF span oceans and continents. It is truly quite inspiring.

It is not hard to understand why a person would turn to alcohol and/or drugs to escape the physical and mental anguish of surviving NF. However, doing so can hurl the already suffering individual into a spiraling depression. Remember: Facing your feelings—no matter how painful—is the only way to overcome them so you can go on with your life. Abusing alcohol and/or drugs only delays—and magnifies—the hard work you alone must do to overcome the emotional fallout of a traumatic event such as surviving NF.

Nightmares and Flashbacks

Even though I saw my open wounds while I was sick, it really didn't have a huge impact on me emotionally. But a couple of years after my experience, I was in my garden, admiring my beautiful crop of tomatoes that I had grown from seed. I reached down to pick up one tomato that had fallen to the ground. I turned it over, and there was a hideous-looking, rotten, gaping hole in it. I was instantly overcome with fear and revulsion: My heart raced, and I felt dizzy. The hole reminded me of my abdomen when I was sick. My emotional reaction took me by surprise. I realized then that I had really gone through something horrific and had squashed the fear down inside me.

—Jacqueline Roemmele

Nightmares and flashbacks like the one just described are not unusual in survivors of a traumatic illness or event. They are the byproduct of the underlying fear and anxiety resulting from one's experience.

Flashbacks are unpredictable and somewhat alarming for many survivors of a traumatic event. Even years later, a sight, sound, or smell may instantly bring you back through time to a memory as clear and multidimensional as if it were actually happening. You may feel an intensity of emotion that you do not recall feeling at the time. Flashbacks and nightmares can also be triggered by events such as the anniversary of your experience with NF or of a loved one's death from the disease.

When a frightening flashback or nightmare occurs, breathe deeply and remind yourself that what you are experiencing is normal after suffering from such a traumatic event and that it will pass. Learning simple relaxation techniques (such as those Irene Koenig describes later in this chapter) can help you regain control after a flashback or nightmare. In addition, talk openly with a loved one or therapist about your experiences. Write in your journal, describing the event in detail.

Emotional Numbness

Is it possible to feel absolutely nothing as you recover from NF, despite the fact that you suddenly find yourself to be an amputee or marred by scars? The answer is yes, but this does not mean that you are devoid of feelings. More likely than not, your brain, with its remarkable ability to protect you from overwelming emotion, has switched into a kind of robot mode—a detached, seemingly emotionless state in which you are temporarily excused from dealing with your anger, frustration, and other emotions associated with your experience with NF and its crushing effects on your life. However, a human being operating in robot mode for an extended period of time is not psychologically healthy and this can have serious physical consequences. Carol Wallace, who we introduced in the last chapter, and who is a certified rehabilitation counselor and an amputee herself, explains why in her book *Challenged by Amputation: Embracing a New Life:*

> When recent amputees act as though everything is okay, I grow concerned, even though this deceptive sentiment is common during the first year following amputation. Not expressing or not feeling anger isn't unusual, yet not doing so can end up causing problems that may show up in other ways, like heart problems, ulcers, headaches, or addictive patterns.

When a patient finally demonstrates that he or she is angry about their amputation, Carol is pleased because she knows that the patient's grieving process has begun.

In order to cope with and eliminate your emotional numbness, spend time alone with your thoughts. Relaxation techniques, meditation, and listening to soothing music in a comfortable, private setting can put you in touch with the reality and intensity of your feelings. Remind yourself that emotions that you may be avoiding, such as depression and anger, are valid, regardless of their nature, and give yourself permission to feel them in order to heal.

Keeping a journal is advice that is often repeated throughout this chapter. Putting thoughts to paper (or computer screen) holds special significance when it comes to breaking out of robot mode and into feeling the normal, healthy emotions of loss. Writing can serve as a catharsis, opening the floodgates of your emotions and unburdening your heart and mind.

Why Me?

There are few human emotions as warm, comforting, and enveloping as self-pity. And nothing is more corrosive and destructive. There is only one answer; turn away from it and move on.

—Dr. Megan Reik

Dr. Reik's advice is sound, but is often much easier said than done. Self-pity is a natural reaction to suffering such a debilitating and life-changing experience. You may wonder what you did to deserve such a cruel twist in your life. You may feel as though you are a victim, and nothing anyone says to you to brighten your outlook can help. As may be the case with depression and anger, living with a person wallowing in self-pity can be taxing on loved ones trying to be as supportive as humanly possible. Self-pity makes one pessimistic, quick to tears, and miserable to be around.

Nevertheless, feeling sorry for oneself is a natural reaction to a life-changing event such as surviving necrotizing fasciitis. Like anger, we must experience our true emotions in order to mend our hearts, spirits, and bodies.

Try to remember to count your blessings. Despite your living with disability or disfigurement, there are many gifts in your life—including the fact that you actually survived NF. Become aware of your blessings: your children, spouse, and friends. Allow yourself to mourn your broken dreams, but then file them away and look for the possibilities and potential in your life. If you have access to the Internet, read the stories of others who have been affected by NF. Through their inspiring words, perhaps you can find some truth and meaning for yourself. Reach out to others whose stories touch you, and accept the comforting shoulder that is offered to you.

Try looking at yourself in a new way! Not as a victim, but as a *victor*. Your scars are like badges of courage, the result of winning the long and painful battle against a microscopic killer. Many others have not been so lucky. As a survivor, you are a testament to what the human body and spirit are capable of overcoming. Talk about your experience from the position of someone who has triumphed over tragedy, and be proud of the example you set for other people to do the same.

Scott Miller, from Helena, Ohio, who spent nearly two months in the intensive care unit fighting NF in 1997, shares his experience:

> Talking about what happened when I was sick with NF has worked best for me throughout my recovery and healing process. At first, when I used to talk about it, I would get a big lump in my throat and tears in my eyes. It now has been two years since it happened to me, and when I talk to people about it now, I get this great feeling of satisfaction and well-being that I have now helped others by educating them about NF.

Acceptance

While the emotions we have just highlighted are common to NF survivors, each survivor is different and will experience his or her own personal journey toward the ultimate goal: acceptance. Acceptance is a "place" in our minds and hearts that, once reached, allows us to go on with our lives relatively intact. We no longer feel debilitated by anger, depression, self-pity, or any other negative emotions. However, reaching a place of acceptance does not mean that you will never have negative feelings, flashbacks, or longings to do the things we used to be able to do. Carol Wallace explains this well:

> To this day, my chest tightens whenever I enter a place with a dance floor. Dancing was one of my favorite activities in the whole world. I was a wonderful dancer and always danced in my high heels. Giving my high heels to Goodwill, knowing I would never again be able to dance the way I used to, still hurts. It's hard to watch other people enjoying what I used to do so well. Fourteen years haven't dimmed my desire to jitterbug or do the twist.

Acceptance can also mean we can laugh about our experience. Author Jacqueline Roemmele quips, "When talking to young children about their NF experiences, I tell them that when I lie on my back, from the way the skin on my abdomen healed, it looks like I have two belly buttons, both 'innies.' My mom used to tease me when I was a little girl that God made innies as a convenient place for salt when you're eating french fries in bed. Well, now I have one for ketchup too."

Paul Fasolas, a bodybuilder, father, and NF survivor from Orlando, Florida, also relies on humor to talk about his experience:

> After five days on a ventilator, I woke up to my wife with her nose in my face saying, "Paul, Paul. You are alive, and everything is going to be all right." Knowing my wife as well as I did, I believed her and was comforted by that. She continued, "We had to take off your left leg to save your life. Do you understand?" I could see my two young sons over her shoulder, and I did understand, because exchanging my leg for the rest of my life with my family seemed like a good deal to me.
>
> Now I have lost her [sadly, Paul's wife died of cancer just a year after Paul's bout with NF], but my sons are the light of my life, and I must continue to set an example for them as well as for others who have suffered from NF. It seems that so many people like my attitude that I get calls from various doctors or surgeons asking me to talk with someone who has recently suffered an amputation, specifically a hip disarticulation [amputation from the hip]. I generally approach them with humor and then get down to the fact that if it had not been for the amputation, they would not be lucky enough to be talking with me. Also, my story seems to make most people feel fortunate.

Acceptance in NF survivors can also lead to a wondrous transformation in one's inner spirituality and one's relationship with God. We'll discuss this common thread in greater detail later in the chapter.

We hope that the guidelines we have provided in these pages will be helpful to readers to understand what to expect after surviving necrotizing fasciitis. It is important to keep in mind that everyone is different, and therefore, everyone will react differently. For some the path to psychological and emotional recovery is much easier when accompanied by a professional guide. In the following pages we will provide a brief overview of some of the traditional and alternative therapies available for survivors of NF.

Conventional Therapy for Psychological Healing

While it's easy to say you must deal with your emotions and get through them in order to begin your emotional and psychological recovery, actually doing this is another story. Coping with the emotional changes inherent in recovering from necrotizing fasciitis is not easy to do alone. It is generally a good idea to seek expert assistance in your psychological and emotional recovery process.

> For the most part, I am very positive and keep moving each and every minute of each day. I do not waste time on petty things and try to use each and every moment wisely. I do feel guilty, though, for yelling at my kids and getting upset with them, considering that they, too, are a gift from God and should be cherished. Survivors *must* move forward. And if you are having a hard time handling your emotions, seek out help immediately! And enjoy your family, your friends, and life! Life is so precious!
>
> —Carol Rolfe

Conventional Psychotherapy

The guidance of a skilled and compassionate psychotherapist, psychologist, or psychiatrist can be a godsend for NF survivors who are having difficulty working through the emotional toll of their experience. Psychotherapists offer a safe environment in which to allow patients to work through their feelings at their own pace. The underlying belief system of psychotherapists varies (Freudian or Jungian, for example), and so it is best to find a psychotherapist with whom you feel comfortable. Some states offer referral services that confidentially interview the prospective patient prior to making a referral to try to match a patient's specific needs and personality with the best possible mental health professional.

Private psychotherapy sessions can be costly and therefore out of reach for people without adequate insurance coverage. If this is the case for you, we encourage you to contact your state health department, which may offer programs for people in need at a very low cost.

Group Therapy

Group therapy can also be effective in helping to overcome the emotions of loss following a traumatic illness such as necrotizing fasciitis. A group consisting of NF survivors would be ideal; however, in many locations, it may be difficult to arrange such a group in light of the rarity of the disease. Therefore, a group consisting of people suffering from any number of traumatic illnesses or life events may be just as beneficial.

The advantages of group therapy are many. The camaraderie and support network that develops among group members can be the catalyst to the psychological and emotional recovery for many people. Group therapy also offers a unique advantage to NF survivors. Dr. Jay Earley, a psychologist and author from Larkspur, California, explains it this way:

> Part of the psychological damage that survivors of necrotizing fasciitis endure can be attributed to the public nature of the disease—the highly visible scarring, amputations, misinformation, etc. NF survivors may be anxious or fearful about how they will be viewed and treated by others. While private, one-on-one therapy sessions are certainly worthwhile in addressing these feelings, the actual sharing and interaction that occurs in the public—but safe—environment of group therapy can prove to be even more valuable.

Antidepressant Drug Therapy

In moderate to severe cases of depression, antidepressant drugs may be helpful for about seven out of ten people. Antidepressants work by targeting the neurotransmitters in the brain that carry chemicals from one cell to the other. In between the cells of the brain are tiny spaces called synapses. The function of the neurotransmitters is to assist the nerve impulses in jumping from one cell to another. Once the nerve impulse has cleared the synapse with the help of the neurotransmitter, an enzyme steps in and sweeps up the neurotransmitter in preparation for the next impulse to come along.

People who are depressed suffer from low levels of certain types of neurotransmitters. Antidepressants work by blocking the enzymes that sweep up neurotransmitters from the synapses between cells, a process known as reuptake inhibition.

Drug therapy is usually prescribed and managed by a psychiatrist. The psychiatrist will prescribe one or more drugs, depending on the patient's symptoms and complaints. Therefore, it is very important that the patient be open and honest about his or her feelings in order for the right type, dosage, and combination of drugs to be prescribed. Typically it takes several weeks for the antidepressant drugs to be effective.

As of this writing, antidepressant drugs such as Prozac (fluoxetine hydrochloride) and Wellbutrin SR (bupropion hydrochloride) are generally considered to be safe and nonaddictive; however, there are side effects. Most commonly, people report dramatic changes in libido. Weight gain or loss, dry mouth, anxiety, nausea, insomnia, drowsiness, tremors, and sweating have also been noted.

While antidepressant drugs can certainly ease depression and elevate the mood of the patient, it is important to remember that the problems that exacerbated depression do not evaporate into thin air once medication is begun. Combining antidepressant medication with psychotherapy can ensure that once the state of depression is lifted, it is not likely to return.

To learn more about prescription medication for depression, contact a qualified psychiatrist in your area.

Alternative Approaches to Psychological Healing

For many of us, the idea of taking psychotropic medication or spending years in psychotherapy sessions in order to cope with the psychological and emotional trauma of NF is unappealing. Thankfully, there are many alternative approaches that can be drug-free, painless, and, surprisingly quick. The key is to find a technique that works for you and a relationship with a clinician who has excellent skills and whom you can trust.

Emotional Freedom Techniques

Emotional Freedom Techniques (EFT) is an alternative, short-term emotional healing method that reduces or resolves trauma as well as anxiety, depression, and most grief reactions. It is also used to enhance positive work and sports performance, among other things.

Its theory is based on the premise that all negative emotions are the result of a disruption in the body's energy system. To explain the EFT method, we spoke to Deborah Mitnick, a psychotherapist and personal performance coach from Baltimore, Maryland, who specializes in EFT as well as other energy-based modalities. Deborah has worked with severe trauma of all types, including surgery and serious illness, armed robberies, sudden deaths, murders and attempted murders, kidnappings, etc. She has also been a crisis interventionist at an emergency room of a Baltimore hospital and has provided grief counseling to both patients and their families. She explains it this way:

> Imagine a TV set working normally. The picture and sound are clear, and the electricity is flowing smoothly. But what would happen if you took the back of the set off and poked a screwdriver through the wires? You would quite obviously disrupt or reroute the flow of electricity and an electric *zzzzt* would occur inside. The picture and sound would lose clarity and the TV would exhibit its version of a "negative emotion.
>
> In the same manner, according to EFT theory, when our

energy systems become imbalanced, we have an electrical *zzzzt* effect going on inside of us. Straighten out this *zzzzt* and the negative emotion goes away. Through EFT we are able to straighten out the energy flow in the body that caused the disruption.

EFT works by having the client "tune into" specific thoughts, feelings, or images of the situation (emotional or physical) that he or she wants to correct, while tapping on specific areas of the body that are sensitive to bioelectrical impulses, similar to the points used in acupressure. It is also often an experience that is relatively free of emotional pain, because the tapping reduces the emotional intensity of the challenge being viewed very quickly.

How does it work? Stimulating these acupressure points by tapping releases endorphins, which are the chemicals that often relieve both physical and emotional pain. As a result, emotional and often physical pain can be reduced or resolved, and the flow of blood and oxygen to the affected area is increased. This causes the muscles to relax, promotes healing, and in effect rebalances the body's energy system. Immediate and dramatic relief is often experienced. The tapping can also dissolve tension and stress, which inhibit the immune system and keep the body from functioning smoothly. Many clients report that they feel better physically after sessions that deal with emotional issues. EFT is highly effective in resolving or greatly reducing traumatic incidence. Deborah and her colleagues report that their clients experience long-term relief.

Deborah tells us:

I use many techniques of energy therapy, including EFT, to promote rapid healing and recovery. While I make no guarantees or promises, often only a few in-office visits or phone sessions are usually needed to clear energy blockages and restore healthy emotional and physical functioning in the specific area that's being addressed. My success rate is in the high 90-percent range for emotional issues and in the high 80-percent range for phys-

Nonprescription Supplements for Depression

The popularity of holistic and natural medicine for treating physical and psychological ailments has soared in recent years. Experts in natural medicine report that vitamin supplementation and herbal remedies can help to alleviate depression without the need for harsh prescriptions. Keeping in mind that it is always best to consult a qualified physician when seeking to treat symptoms of depression, let's explore some of these natural remedies.

St. John's Wort

St. John's wort, or *Hypericum perforatum,* which can be purchased just about anywhere, has become all the rage for self-treating mild to moderate depression. According to some recently published clinical studies, St. John's wort (*wort* is from the Old English terminology for root, herb, or plant) is living up to the hype as an excellent natural alternative to prescription antidepressants. St. John's wort is new only to the United States, however. European countries, especially Germany, consider St. John's wort a quite effective remedy for treating anxiety, depression, and sleep disorders. Doctors in European countries and write tens of millions of prescriptions for this herbal supplement per year—twice as often as for prescription antidepressants such as Prozac.

The advantages of this herbal remedy, according to reports, include far fewer side effects than prescription antidepressants, particularly sexual dysfunction.

Ginseng

Ginseng is one of the most popular medicinal herbs in the world, dating back over 4,000 years. Siberian ginseng has been recorded throughout Chinese history as a memory enhancer. Recent research also demonstrates that ginseng improves blood flow to the brain, allowing serotonin levels to rise, which in turn, has a positive effect on depression.

Ginkgo Biloba

Also an extremely popular and ancient medicinal supplement, *Ginkgo biloba* is made from the leaves of the tree bearing the same name. *Ginkgo biloba* also affects serotonin, it is reported, by increasing the number of serotonin receptor sites on brain cells, which decrease as we grow older, hence, alleviating depression.

L-Tyrosine

According to Dr. James F. Balch in his book *Prescription for Nutritional Healing,* L-tyrosine, a multifunction amino acid, is instrumental in regulating mood, among its other important functions, such as mitigating the appetite and assisting in the reduction of body fat. A deficiency of L-tyrosine can directly lead to depression. Dr. Balch recommends taking L-tyrosine in conjunction with 50 milligrams of vitamin B$_6$ and 100 to 500 milligrams of vitamin C at bedtime. People taking MAO inhibitors, prescription antidepressant drugs, must not take L-tyrosine supplements.

L-tyrosine is found naturally in almonds, avocados, bananas, dairy products, lima beans, pumpkin seeds, and sesame seeds.

Certain Vitamin Supplements

Many physicians believe that certain vitamin deficiencies can lead to or intensify emotional distress, including depression. Be sure that you are getting enough of the following vitamins:

- **Vitamin B$_6$.** According to reports, as little as 10 milligrams of vitamin B$_6$ per day can alleviate depression.
- **Folic acid.** Several reports have reported that folic acid levels are low in individuals who are depressed.
- **Vitamin C.** Insufficient amounts of this important vitamin can result in depression.

ical issues. I've worked with many people who have spent years in conventional psychotherapy sessions without achieving the results they were looking for. With EFT, emotional issues are generally easily resolved. Many of my colleagues who practice energy therapies have also reported significant remissions in other conditions, including chronic pain, stress, arthritis, lupus, allergies, the *symptoms* of multiple sclerosis, HIV, chronic fatigue, low self esteem, sinus problems, diabetes, addictions, athletic performance, anger, and habit control.

In her role as a personal performance coach, Deborah offers telephone consultations and practices EFT worldwide. To learn more about emotional freedom techniques, see the Resources section of this book.

Traumatic Incident Reduction

Developed by Yale- and Stanford-trained psychiatrist Frank A. Gerbode, Traumatic Incident Reduction (TIR) is a brief, one-on-one, nonhypnotic, person-centered, highly structured method for eliminating the negative effects of past traumas. It involves a facilitator, someone specifically trained in TIR techniques, to guide the client through the repeated viewing of a specific traumatic memory from a third-person point of view. It is as if the client is watching the event unfold on videotape. TIR is performed under safe conditions that minimize distractions. Sessions are not limited to the conventional fifty-minute hour; the client is permitted as much session time as she needs to reach a point of resolution or comfort.

"A trauma stays 'stuck' because we often tend to want to push the memories of a specific trauma away from our thoughts. Such is the nature of post-traumatic stress disorder," Deborah Mitnick, also a practitioner of TIR, explains. "But if we attempt to repress the trauma, it often manifests in negative physical and emotional symptoms. However, if we can *embrace* the trauma, we can neutralize it, along with most, if not all of the destructive effects it has on the mind and body."

While TIR may seem more confrontational and frightening than the relatively "painless" EFT, the client only views what he is comfortable with during the session. After several runs through of the traumatic event, the client usually becomes more courageous in contacting his or her emotions as well as the details of the event. By repeatedly viewing the event in the safety and structure of the TIR session, the event usually becomes neutralized. Just as with EFT, the memories of the trauma are not forgotten; in fact, they may even become clearer. It's the emotional intensity of the event that often melts away.

Deborah tells us, "The feedback I receive from my clients indicates that TIR often leads to clients' increased ability to function, elimination of nightmares and flashbacks, enhanced relationships, and a greater sense of empowerment and contentment."

For more information about Traumatic Incident Reduction, see the Resources section of this book.

Spiritual Recovery

There are those of us who have reached a place where we have been blessed with a special understanding of humanity. I think we reach this place when something traumatic occurs in our lives. This trauma opens up a dormant part of our spiritual abilities. Without the trauma we would probably go along in our ho-hum way and never come to realize a whole other part of our "humanness."

> —Diana Cahill, mother of Matthew, 17, who died
> of NF complicated by streptococcal toxic shock
> syndrome

Recovering from a severe illness like NF or unexpectedly losing someone dear to us changes us forever. Suddenly it seems that people around us are consumed by insignificant day-to-day problems, not realizing how precious life is and how quickly it can be taken away. Soul-searching, or looking within ourselves to find the meanings of and lessons in our experience, as well as connecting to a loving, overseeing power for strength and guidance, becomes integral to our daily lives—

and can be extremely beneficial to the overall healing process. In this section, we'll talk about the spiritual aspect of recovering from the NF experience. As often as possible, we share the personal, inspiring, and sometimes miraculous stories from survivors or surviving loved ones.

The Power of Prayer

No matter what the religion, system of belief, or culture, prayer is the universal healer and one of the most essential ingredients to developing our inner selves. We can pray for healing, peace, justice, love, truth, God's will, and more. While suffering from NF, prayer for one's survival can unite family, friends, and strangers across the miles. And as you recover, prayer can be invaluable to finding the personal meaning in your experience and your ability to cope with our physical, psychological, and spiritual recovery.

Irene Koenig, a holistic counselor, teacher, and Pathwork helper practicing in Connecticut and Massachusetts, explains, "Creating your own prayer can be of tremendous assistance throughout the healing process. You may pray for help in understanding and accepting your situation. Pray to open yourself up to spiritual assistance—as well as the assistance of your fellow human beings right here on earth. Pray to be held safely by your doctors and those who help facilitate your healing process. Pray to be guided in your choices. You will feel less alone on your healing journey. Invite God to be with you."

Irene crafted the following prayer as an example for NF survivors.

Dear God,
Thank you for this day.
I pray for help in accepting this disease.
I pray for the humility to accept your will.
I ask for help to love myself in my imperfection; to find my way
    as I move through the healing process.
I pray to open myself to receiving your guidance to know ways
    to help myself.
I pray for help in accepting this disease.

I ask to be sent healers and helpers along the way to help me
through my healing process.
I ask for your help to recognize them.
I open myself to be guided by love.
I pray that I may love myself.
I pray for others with this disease.
Thank you, God.
Amen.

Contemplating God's Role in the NF Experience

Necrotizing fasciitis is a swift and deadly infection. The cruelty of the
disease can make us, understandably, question God's intentions. How
could He allow us—or someone we love—to suffer in such a horrible
way? Or, we may find ourselves thanking God every day of our lives for
his divine intervention in allowing us or someone we love to survive
against all odds.

Regardless of religious affiliation, turning to God gives NF victims
and their families inner strength to get through the darkest hours of the
illness when there is nothing else that medical science can do for the patient. We are aware of many patients for whom there have been all-night
prayer vigils, worldwide prayer lines uniting friends and strangers alike,
and family and friends holding hands and praying around the bed. How
often we hear, "It was only through prayer and God's will that I survived!" Even when the unthinkable happens, when someone dies from
his or her battle with NF, it is often the faith that the individual is in
heaven that comforts the grieving family.

In the following paragraphs, we share the personal experience of NF
survivors or surviving family members.

I was utterly devastated when my husband, Arney, died from
NF after open-heart surgery. Arney's career was as an electrical
inspector, which he loved. The day of Arney's burial, the
church in which we were having the service was the only
building in town that had no power. The ONLY building! I
clearly remember Father Michael, a close friend of ours, be-

ginning his eulogy in the dark. "If ever we could use Arney's skills, it would be right now," he said. As soon as those words left Father Michael's mouth, the lights in the church came on with a flourish. The many mourners, friends, and family who filled the pews gasped. And despite my grief, inside my heart, I smiled: Arney was telling us in his own special way that he was still with us.

—Ann Marie Robertson, about her
husband, Arnold, Massachusetts

Besides the mid-thigh amputation, between June of 1996 and March of 1998 I have had a colostomy, two major skin grafts, and five reconstructive surgeries on my lower back. I have had thirty-eight major operations since 1980, survived two pulmonary embolisms and a cardiac arrest, and, because of my multiple sclerosis, am also paraplegic. No one knows how I contracted NF, but the fact that I have MS may explain why it was so severe. I have absolutely no doubt that God intervened and preserved my life, and I am joined in that belief by several hard-bitten and normally skeptical doctors.

—Doug Fitzpatrick, California (Doug later learned to ski despite his
pain and injuries. The quote he lives by, quite successfully, is Winston Churchill's: "Never give in! Never, never, never, never, never
give in!")

My partner, my wife, wasn't there anymore, I knew that God had relieved her of this pain, and she had already put on her heavenly garments and left this world behind. As her blood pressure dropped and the emotional numbness took hold of me, I met with family and friends and encouraged everyone as best I could and didn't try to hide my tears. A song that I heard after all of this came to me: "Sometimes He calms the storm, and sometimes He calms His child." I am sure He was with me during these tough hours, all through the "storm."

I napped with the kids in a small room. At 3:30 A.M. on the twenty-third of December, I awoke and knew it was time to let

The Miracle of Matthew and Grant

⑥

We have been touched by so many uplifting stories from NF survivors or the loved ones of those who have died from all over the world since the inception of our foundation in early 1997. Of the thousands of people who have contacted us, the story and spiritual connection between Matthew Cahill and Grant Drummond stands out as one of the most extraordinary and heartwarming we have ever received.

In June of 1998, Matthew was a happy, active and popular seventeen-year-old. He was an honors student who loved sailing, swimming, and being a lifeguard. His dream was to become a police officer. Without warning, however, Matthew contracted a violent case of NF complicated by streptococcal toxic shock syndrome that may have entered his body through a fungal infection in his toe, although this has never been confirmed. Matthew's toenail was surgically removed in the late afternoon of Wednesday, June 10. On Friday, June 12, his illness became apparent. Early that evening, his fever reached 107 degrees. Upon visiting a local walk-in clinic, the attending doctor diagnosed Matthew as having flulike symptoms. His recommendation was to give him Tylenol and that if he didn't improve in the morning, to then go to the local emergency room. Unfortunately, Matthew claimed he felt better on the morning of June 13. Sadly, as the day progressed, he took a dramatic turn for the worse until finally it became painfully apparent he was deathly ill. An ambulance was called and he was rushed to emergency. Despite the best efforts by a team of top-notch physicians, Matthew died from heart failure while in surgery.

The community of Kingston, Ontario, was devastated over the sudden loss of Matthew. Over 400 people were present at his memorial service, at which Kingston Ontario Provincial Police officers, in full uniform, served as pallbearers. His parents, Martin and Diana; Matthew's former Sea Scout leader, Lorne Dudley; and his Grandpa Simpson held a service for Matthew on Lorne's sailboat on the Thursday after his funeral. His ashes were scattered in Lake Ontario near Brothers Island.

Unbeknownst to the Cahills and their friends, another man lay fighting for his life in a Toronto hospital. Forty-three-year-old Grant Drummond, a husband and father of two young boys, struggled to beat the 10-percent chance he was given to live. Soon after the debridement of the flesh under his left arm, he went into a coma. His family watched as his hands and feet turned black before them. Group A strep had sent his body into war against itself. He had gone into complete renal failure. If he made it through the night, his family was assured that he would likely require both kidneys transplanted and he would lose both hands and feet. He lay motionless for ten days in his coma, hooked up to sixteen IV lines, respirator, and dialysis.

Ann Perry, Grant's sister, remembers it well: "We received a call in my Halifax home on Sunday, June twenty-third. Grant had only minutes left to live and then he would suffer a heart attack and die. We were told not to come to the hospital, as no one had time. I called my oldest brother, Ross, in Kingston, Ontario, and I told him that Grant would be gone very shortly. He went off to his church in Kingston to pray for Grant."

That same Sunday morning, Martin and Diana attended Syndenham United Church for the first time. Ross introduced himself to Martin and Diana and told them that he knew only too well the pain they were suffering, as his brother was fighting the same battle with NF as they spoke. Diana promised to pray for Grant's recovery.

Diana explains, "That evening, I had a talk with Matthew. I asked him to find Grant in his spiritual travels. I asked him to give Grant the strength and the will to fight for his life. 'Don't let this horrible disease take another life like it took yours. . . . Get in there and make sure it doesn't claim another victim!'"

Meanwhile, in Halifax, Grant's sister Ann called a prayer line in the United States. She cried as she asked for God's will in the matter of her brother. Devastated and exhausted, she wept until she fell asleep. The next morning, much to her surprise, Ann awoke full of confidence, her heart bursting with hope. Reaching for Grant's picture, she told him that she wasn't sure why, but she just knew he was going to be fine. It was a feeling she would never forget. Ann believed that she received a divine gift—a visit from an angel—during the night of June 23, and she was assured that Grant would survive.

And yet, Grant's family was never given any hope whatsoever that he would survive. Eleven weeks after the onset of his bout with NF, his heart stopped three times in one day. He suffered a horrifying brain seizure that went on for over four minutes. He had lost 70 percent of his oxygen to his brain for over twenty minutes, and it was expected he would more than likely be severely mentally impaired if by some miracle he pulled through. His MRI showed what was described as the worst MRI the chief neurologist had ever seen.

Amazingly, however, to the shock and delight of the medical staff, Grant woke up twenty-four hours later and started asking very intelligent questions! This, coming from a man who had died five times in the past several weeks! Completely beating the odds, Grant's internal organs healed as strong as ever, and he suffered no brain damage at all! His hands and feet, once black and destined to be amputated, returned to normal. The entire medical staff declared Grant's recovery a miracle! Grant was eventually released to recuperate at home.

It was early November when Ann went to the National Necrotizing Fasciitis Foundation (NNFF) Web site, where she read an entry in the guest book from Diana, who had shared the story of her son's life and death. Ann cautiously wrote a supportive letter to her telling her how sorry she was for her loss—but to be encouraged that angels really do exist because she had had the pleasure of meeting one during Grant's battle with NF. She assured Diana that Matthew was an angel in heaven looking out for his family.

Nothing could have prepared Ann for the letter that would follow from Diana the next day. Diana informed Ann that she had indeed prayed to Matthew to help Grant. Ann was overwhelmed. Intuitively she knew it was Matthew who had come to her during the night of June twenty-third, but to be absolutely sure, she had to know when Mathew died. Was it June? July? August? Her curiosity prevailed, and so she wrote back to Diana, only to discover that Matthew had died only ten days before Diana had sent her prayers to her son for Grant. They soon discovered that June twenty-third not only was the day that Ann felt the divine intervention by her angel visit, but it was also the day Diana sent her prayers to Matthew for help! Matthew was indeed the angel Ann had met that night!

Diana responded to Ann by saying, "Your letter let me know that Matthew heard me, and with the combined efforts of prayer, medicine, and Grant's own will, he was given back to your family. After I read your letter, I said thanks to Matthew. I feel deep in my soul that God just couldn't deny his newest angel's request: Please give this man back to his family."

Ann and Diana continue to exchange miles of heartfelt letters. They have become true kindred spirits—joined by an experience that will forever mark their souls.

---

her body go. The family prayed in the hall, then I went in to say good-bye to Pamela. As I stroked her hair and spoke of her life and how I would miss her, her "life" glided from this body, smoothly and gently, safely and comfortably—this world was finished for her. It was 4:35 A.M. on December 23, 1995. I sat with her for a few hours without machines on or hurried activities all around, I wanted to feel her peace and her presence. I always loved watching Pamela sleep, only now I knew she would awaken in a place full of greater love that we can experience here.

—Steven A. Berkemeier, about his wife, Pamela

The last three months have been a life-changing experience. I went through a lot of emotions and thoughts I never knew I would. I never thought I would be angry with God, but I was. I never thought I would not trust God, and at times I didn't. I never thought I would believe God would let us suffer, but it happened.

I prayed and begged God to help us. And at the moments when Stephanie was at her worst and we needed Him most, I couldn't feel Him anymore. I found it very hard to pray. I couldn't turn Stephanie over to Him because I was afraid of what He would do to her. At one point, when I should have grabbed for God, I felt that maybe He was the cause for all of this. I believed before that God could heal us. If we got sick and prayed, God had it within His power to take the sickness away; after all, He is God. But as I sat there watching Stephanie suffer and almost die several different times, I decided it may not be the way things work. How could God intentionally allow Stephanie to suffer this way for so long? How could He allow Ann and I to suffer and worry this way?

But after reflecting on Stephanie's experience, I have come to believe that Stephanie simply got a bad germ that did a lot of damage. Stephanie fought it, and she won. I no longer feel angry at God.

—Terrill Sebastian, about his daughter, Stephanie

Meditation for Spiritual Recovery

Meditation is a devotional exercise of reflection and contemplation. It is used as part of every major religion in one degree or another. Many researchers believe that meditation can have positive effects on health, including alleviating depression, anxiety, and chronic pain. Meditation can also help one find personal meaning in his or her own experience, as well as cope with the physical, psychological, and social impact of the disease. Meditating is not difficult, and the results can be calming, self-assuring, uplifting, and spiritually satisfying. Renowned author and spiritual teacher Eva Pierrachos created a method of personal purification and transformation called the Pathwork, which is detailed in her book, *The Pathwork of Self-Transformation* (Bantam). She has also written 257 lectures on spiritual growth. In the lectures, Eva states that there are many meditation practices. We meditate to be in stillness, to positively create our life through eliminating negativity. Through meditation, we can establish contact with our higher wisdom, bring out our positive and creative tendencies, and open ourselves to receive God's help.

We asked Irene Koenig, who we introduced earlier in this chapter, to describe some of the fundamental steps to meditation that she teaches to both individuals and groups. She explains:

> There are different postures and practices of meditation. Here is one example: Create a relaxing, peaceful atmosphere. If you wish, light a candle and/or have soothing music playing softly in the background. Have writing paper and a pen available. Sit in a comfortable chair and place your hands on your thighs, palms up. This is a receptive and open position. Take deep breaths through your nose and out through your mouth, quieting yourself. Then breathe normally.
>
> Begin by clearly formulating and stating your intentions for the meditation. For example, *I want to be able to express my feelings about my experience with NF.* Repeat this statement to yourself clearly. Sit in silence. If negative thoughts arise regarding this intention, you can write about them on your paper. Through writing, you empty out your negative thoughts about what you want. Afterward, come back to your intention for the meditation. In order to create something in our lives, it is important to visualize what we want. Visualize yourself freely expressing your feelings. Picture yourself openly expressing yourself. You are picturing an achievable outcome. Wait in a mindset of faith that this can and will happen. In effect, you are creating a state of being that opens you to bringing about the fulfillment of your intention. Most important, if meditation is difficult for you, be easy with yourself. Its purpose is to help you.

NF and Self-Awakening

Many NF survivors believe that experiencing a traumatic illness can be spiritually self-awakening, resulting in a transformation of priorities, attitudes, and goals. As you work through your emotional responses to your situation, you become more in tune with what is truly important in your life: family, true friendships, compassion, and love. You may even find your true life's mission.

"Surviving NF can be a lonely journey because the damage to our bodies makes us want to hide—even from ourselves, which can be very painful," explains Irene Koenig. "We need to learn to love and accept our bodies through the healing process. We may have to release pride that says you must look a certain way. This may mean embracing the values of *being* versus *appearance*. Letting go of concern of how people view our scars and deformities will bring about self-confidence. As you connect and awaken to the profound knowledge of your real self, you will experience a deep inner security.

"It does not mean that you will never be hurt or affected by others. When security is based on who you are inside, how others view you will not shake your foundation. Operating from the truth of your inner being is a solid foundation from which to live your life."

As hard as it is to believe, most find that their brush with death and what they have undergone serves to enhance their lives. It makes people take time to find new skills or new appreciation for the things in their life, to spend more time with their families, and to find out what they are really made of.

For instance, author Jacqueline Roemmele admits, "I used to commute two and a half hours each way every day, back and forth to a job I thought was the most important thing in the world. My experience with NF grounded me. Who knows what track I'd be on if NF hadn't involuntarily stopped me and put me on another path?"

Author Donna Batdorff felt a "calling" because of her experience with NF. "I remember lying in the hospital thinking, 'Why?'—not as in 'why me?' but more like, 'why did I survive, why was I chosen to have this rare affliction? What am I to do with this?' I had the sense that I had been chosen to survive because I was the type of person to deal with it, and then take the message to other people. "It can be a burden to suddenly have a calling, because you have no choice but to follow it." But interestingly, like Jackie, Donna's career path has included journalism, promotion, and public relations. "I think all of these talents were preparing me for what I would need to do to promote NF awareness and help others."

We recommend the movie *Regarding Henry,* which starred Harrison Ford, as a wonderful depiction of how a traumatic event can completely transform the human spirit.

Life after NF is a personal journey that integrates a myriad of physical, psychological, social, and spiritual components. The permanent changes in our bodies can lead us through the full gamut of our emotions, test our inner strength to the limits, and shake our faith in God. Survivors of NF speak of their lives "before NF" and "after NF." The experience often serves as a catalyst for spiritual awakening, making us realize that we are blessed, regardless of our new physical challenges and painful memories.

Our next chapter will address what each of us can do in the home, workplace, and community to promote awareness of NF while learning how to protect ourselves and our families from invasive bacteria.

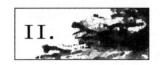

II.

Awareness and Prevention: What You Can Do in the Home, School, and Workplace

⑥

As of this writing, there is no guaranteed way to prevent necrotizing fasciitis from occurring. Perhaps in the years to come, with the approval and release of group A strep vaccines that we discussed in Chapter 7, invasive infections caused by group A strep bacteria will become a disease of the past.

With that in mind, this chapter will focus on what we can do now through awareness and preventive measures to decrease the risk of contracting and spreading bacteria that can result in NF. We'll discuss general methods that apply to everyone, followed by practical suggestions specific to the home, school, and workplace. Expanding further into preventive measures, we'll also discuss some of the products available on the market today that offer some means of personal protection against infectious microorganisms.

General Precautions

There are practical methods of minimizing the possibility of transferring or contracting NF bacteria that apply to everyone. The common themes for this section—indeed, for this entire chapter—are "common sense and courtesy" and "commitment to behavior modification."

If You Have Strep Throat

Strep throat can be the source of an invasive group A strep infection. If you have strep throat symptoms, be responsible and get tested immediately. As disruptive as it is to your life, stay home until you are advised you are no longer contagious. The same applies to your children or other family members. If a child or spouse tests positive for strep throat, it is possible that you (and other household members) will also be carrying the bacteria, with or without symptoms. Although it is not mandatory, you may wish to ask your doctor to test you also for the bacteria. If you also test positive, stay home for the entire time that your physician instructs to ensure that you are no longer in danger of infecting anyone else. Be sure to take the entire course of antibiotics as prescribed.

If You Are Coughing and Sneezing

NF bacteria are transported on respiratory droplets and propelled through the air by coughing and sneezing. While we cannot call in sick to work or stay home from school with every sniffle, it is important to rule out a strep infection if symptoms are suspicious. In any case, the key is to behave consistently as if you could be carrying potentially dangerous bacteria and guide your actions accordingly. Immediately throw out used tissues, and never use fabric handkerchiefs that you sneeze or cough into and then put back in your pocket. Wash your hands after coughing or sneezing into them and before touching anyone or anything. Consider using alcohol-based germ-killing gels and hand wipes as an added precaution.

If You Have an Open Wound

As annoying as it may be, care for each scratch and cut diligently. Wash thoroughly and cover with a new adhesive bandage. Be on the lookout for signs of infection: swelling, redness, pain, and drainage or pus. If symptoms worsen or a fever develops, seek medical treatment immediately.

Awareness and Prevention in the Home

Each of us has a wonderful opportunity to teach awareness and prevention of NF in the home as an integral part of family life. The added benefit is that instilling good habits that can minimize the risk of NF can also reduce the risk of contracting any other type of infection. Here are some smart ways to incorporate NF awareness and prevention in your home:

Call a Family Meeting

Calling a family meeting signals to family members that the subject matter to be discussed is important and will require each person's full attention. Now, those of us with children know that the attention span of youngsters is fleeting, so it is a good idea to keep the meeting brief and to the point.

You can begin by expressing your concerns about invasive bacteria. Perhaps you can describe a specific incident that stands out in your mind, such as a recent NF case in your hometown, and explain that you would never want your family to suffer such a horrible experience. With that said, point out specific situations in which family members are currently engaging in at-risk behavior, such as neglecting injuries or coughing without covering the mouth. Have children think of and share other situations as well.

Then explain the new rules of the household, including washing hands, bringing cuts and scratches to Mom's and Dad's attention, being courteous with sneezes and coughs, etc. As enthusiastic as each family member may be at the time, changing existing behaviors requires follow-up and reinforcement for it to be adopted by each family member, especially children. Teach older children basic injury protocol, such as washing the injury and covering it with an adhesive bandage. Inform each family member about "red-alarm" symptoms (fever, swelling, and pain) that must immediately be brought to the attention of Mom or Dad.

If Your Child Has Chickenpox

As children with chickenpox are members of a high-risk group for contracting the bacteria that cause NF, be vigilant for signs of redness, fever, or pain after the onset of chickenpox. Bring children with suspicious symptoms to the pediatrician or emergency room immediately and ask that the possibility of NF be ruled out. In younger children, it may be helpful to put mittens on little hands to prevent them from scratching at the pox sores, which may reopen the wounds or introduce invasive bacteria into the area.

If Your Child Has Strep Throat

As nowadays both parents in many families work outside the home, having a child suddenly become ill with strep throat can really throw a monkey wrench into our busy lives. Many employers are less than understanding when an employee calls in at the last minute because he or she must stay home with a sick child. Other parents, who absolutely cannot miss work, are tempted to send the child to school if symptoms are mild enough, hoping that the child will get better during the day. However, if your child is suffering from a confirmed case of strep throat, he or she must stay home from school for the twenty-four-hour period following the start of antibiotics in order to minimize the risk of infecting other people, one of whom may develop an invasive infection. Likewise, if your child is in day care with other children, he or she should certainly be kept home until no longer contagious. This holds true for children who are cared for by elderly grandparents, who could be put in jeopardy if caring for a child with strep throat. Furthermore, as we mentioned earlier, if there are other children in the household, it is wise to have them also tested and treated for strep throat, as it is likely to be passed around the family.

As with children with chickenpox, be mindful of the symptoms of an invasive infection in your child with strep throat. Monitor fever, complaints of limb pain, diarrhea, vomiting, or dehydration. Examine the child for reddened, painful areas that are unusual, and immediately seek medical treatment from a reliable physician, voicing your concerns about NF.

Awareness and Prevention in School

Strep throat, the flu, and other illnesses are easily passed from one student to another in schools, sometimes resulting in a large percentage of the students being out sick at one time. While it may be virtually impossible to contain contagious illnesses, there are some commonsense ground rules that parents, teachers, and school nurses can establish in order to minimize disruption and decrease the chances of students contracting invasive infections.

Parents

As difficult as it may be to enforce, teach your children to be courteous and careful at school and in the playground about sniffling, sneezing, coughing, and wiping noses with hands. Encourage frequent hand washing and include kid-size alcohol-based germ-killing gels or wipes in lunches or backpacks.

Furthermore, if your child has symptoms of strep throat but is asking to go to school, err on the side of caution: Have strep throat ruled out before sending the child back to the classroom, where he or she can infect other students. If strep throat is confirmed, ensure that the child is kept home for the full twenty-four-hour period after starting antibiotics to ensure that he or she is no longer contagious.

School Administrators

School administrators should consider establishing policies and procedures for dealing with cases of strep throat, just as they do with chickenpox in many states. It is a good idea to send home a fact sheet about strep throat with students, including its symptoms, complications, and the potential for causing invasive infections such as necrotizing fasciitis. This is in addition to the school's policy about parental responsibility in keeping children home until they are no longer contagious. In doing this, parents are informed about the dangers of strep and are guided in their actions if and when their child becomes ill.

If a child in the school contracts a case of necrotizing fasciitis, many parents will understandably become alarmed about the risk to their own children and look to the school administrators to ease their concerns. Administrators can take a proactive role in disseminating factual information about NF in the wake of a case by holding a special meeting with parents or sending home information with students. A hotline for more information can be established with a responsible authority on the disease.

Teachers

Teachers, especially health and/or science teachers, can make a tremendous contribution to the awareness of NF by including the disease (and others) as part of the curriculum. No matter what the educational level, elementary through high school, learning about diseases and conducting research projects individually or as a group can be quite interesting for students. Studying the dangers of invasive infections also causes youngsters to assess their own at-risk behavior while arming themselves with knowledge of preventive measures and symptoms to watch for.

School Nurses

A school nurse equipped with knowledge of the symptoms, manifestations, and extraordinary speed of invasive infections such as NF can potentially save a child's life by recommending immediate and aggressive medical attention for suspicious symptoms. As far as prevention and awareness, the school nurse can also ensure diligent adherence to the school policy of having children with strep throat stay home as instructed. It is a good idea to establish this policy, as well as others, in writing, with occasional reminders in the school newsletter or in flyers sent home with students.

Awareness and Prevention in the Workplace

Employers can find themselves in a difficult position in that sick employees cost money and interfere with the pace of business. On the other hand, employers must recognize the fact that an employee sick with strep throat who has not been treated can easily pass the illness to others, resulting in several people calling in sick, versus just the one. As a preventive measure, employers should be flexible in allowing employees who complain of strep throat symptoms to get tested and treated as soon as possible.

If an Employee Has Been Diagnosed with NF

A sudden case of NF in the workplace has been known to cause near-mutiny among workers who fear becoming infected. This is understandable and needs to be addressed calmly and assertively by company management. Because company officials are more than likely unfamiliar with the nature of invasive infections, accurate information must be gathered prior to making any public statements to employees. Such information can be obtained through public health agencies and resources such as this book.

Like school administrators, employers should explain that an employee has been diagnosed with necrotizing fasciitis, and that while this is extremely upsetting, there is no need for panic. While it is unlikely that anyone in the office or work environment is in danger of also contracting the disease, employers can make the suggestion that employees with suspicious symptoms (such as strep throat, severe limb pain, and fever) seek treatment. In addition, while reinforcing the fact that invasive bacteria are not likely to be lingering around the workplace, employers can ease any residual concerns by disinfecting multiple-use telephones, doorknobs, restrooms, and other common areas.

Protecting Yourself from Potentially Dangerous Bacteria in the Workplace

Working in close contact with other people can easily expose one to colds, flu, and other potentially dangerous and invasive germs. While we cannot fully protect ourselves from the possibility of becoming sick, there are certain preventive behaviors that can be implemented to considerably lessen our chances.

- If you work in the service industry (handling food or money, working directly with people, etc.), wash your hands frequently and keep a germ-killing alcohol-based agent close at hand. If you have open cuts, abrasions, patches of dermatitis, etc., this is especially important. If feasible, wear gloves.

- If you work in construction, maintenance, landscaping, carpentry, or any profession in which daily cuts, bruises, and scratches are common, be diligent about wearing gloves or, at the very least, washing hands often and caring for cuts and scratches.
- If you work in health care, frequent hand washing can be extremely effective in minimizing the risk of contracting (and spreading) dangerous bacteria. Wear gloves and masks as necessary around sick people, and change gloves between visits.
- If you work with children, keeping the environment as clean as possible, in addition to washing your hands frequently and using antiseptic gels and wipes, can go a long way toward protecting yourself from potentially dangerous bacteria.
- If you work in an office, also wash your hands frequently, and wipe down telephones, headsets, keyboards, etc., that are shared with other employees. Shaking hands also transfers germs from one person to another. If you can't avoid it in your position, be diligent about hand cleanliness to minimize risk.

If You're Sick, Stay Home!

Everyone knows someone like this: a stubborn but well-meaning employee who is sick but insists on working unless he or she is literally falling over in his or her chair. While these people may feel that they are proving their loyalty and dedication to the company, they are doing no one any favors by allowing their germs to be spread all over the workplace. It is inconvenient and sometimes next to impossible, but if you are sick with strep throat, you are putting yourself and others in danger. Get treated and stay home until you are sure that you cannot infect anyone else.

The same advice applies to parents with children who are sick at home with strep throat. Even if you feel perfectly fine and have no symptoms, it may be wise to get tested: It could save someone's life. In fact, sadly enough, a health care worker at an East Coast hospital who was carrying group A strep innocently infected three people she treated, one of whom died. She had absolutely no symptoms; however, it was discovered that her young child was at home suffering from strep throat.

Awareness and Prevention in Special Circumstances

There are often unavoidable circumstances in which you must remain in close quarters with sick individuals, and you may feel somewhat powerless and frightened that you are in danger of contracting an invasive illness. Let's list some of these circumstances and address what can be done to protect our families and ourselves:

- Airplanes
- Crowds (sporting events, church, parades, etc.)
- Gyms
- Elevators
- Hospital or physician waiting rooms
- Public restrooms
- Subways, trains, and other public transportation

There are levels of concern about contracting invasive bacteria that range from nonexistent to informed awareness to extreme pathophobia—a psychological fear of contracting diseases. Most of us fall into the nonexistent-to-informed–awareness category, in which standing in a crowd at a hockey game or in a crowded elevator does not cause us severe anxiety. However, knowing that invasive bacteria are transferred in the respiratory droplets from one person to another or from direct contact with another person, caution and courtesy should guide our actions. Be sure your immune system is in the best possible condition to fight off disease. If someone is coughing or sneezing incessantly behind you, move to another location if at all possible. If you are sick with strep throat, be responsible and avoid public events altogether until you are no longer contagious. Keep your hands clean, and avoid touching public doors, handles, buttons, railings, etc.

The added security of germicidal and air filtering products in the home and/or office may appeal to many people as a means of further lessening the chances of contracting invasive bacteria. Let's cover two of these innovative products.

HEPA Filters

HEPA, which stands for *high-efficiency particulate arresting,* is a popular method of purifying the air of the home or office. According to reports, HEPA filters are capable of removing over 98 percent of bacteria, pollen, mold spores, animal hair and dander, dust, and other airborne particles. There are several types of HEPA filters available at varying sizes and prices.

Personal Air Purifiers

Personal air purifiers, which are about the same weight and size as the average pager, are receiving excellent reviews of their ability to remove bacteria, allergens, and other pollutants from one's personal breathing space. The device is worn around the neck or is placed in the chest pocket. Unfiltered air is drawn in, purified through ionization, and then redirected toward the mouth and nose of the user at a rate consistent with normal breathing.

⑥

While incorporating preventive measures into your life is wise, excessive fear about contracting a deadly disease like NF is unnecessary and immobilizing. The best advice is to establish consistent ground rules in your home, for your children, and in your workplace to be cautious and courteous in the ways we described in this chapter.

Getting the Word Out

The Kingston community is much better informed now because of Matt. He didn't die without purpose or cause. The medical community is much better educated and prepared to handle cases of NF now, much more so than a year ago. Their skills at diagnosing NF are tremendously enhanced now after dealing with numerous cases in the Kingston area . . . the catalyst being Matt back in June of 1998.

—Diana Cahill, Kingston, Ontario

When NF strikes, the horrific nature of the disease, as well as the scarcity of information about it, motivates survivors and surviving family members to ask, "What can I do to help to get the word out?" Here are some excellent suggestions inspired by some incredible people we have met through the foundation:

- Write letters to your public health department, state representatives, local hospitals, etc., about your experience, including information regarding the disease to promote greater awareness and education.
- Contact the National Necrotizing Fasciitis Foundation, Surviving Strep—Strategies for Survival, an organization based in Ontario and founded by a survivor of NF and STSS, Catherine Mulvale, or the Lee Spark NF Foundation in the UK. All three organizations are actively recruiting volunteers for a wide range of activities including community outreach, fundraising, support, etc.
- Write your story and publish it on a personal Web page, or submit it to the NNFF for publication. The World Wide Web is an incredible means of communication and education, and by using it you will be sure to touch many lives.
- Organize fundraising events in remembrance of your child, spouse, or parent who died of NF. Martin and Diana Cahill have begun a wonderful tribute to their son, Matthew, whom they lost to NF/STSS in June of 1998, in conjunction with the family of another Kingston boy, Frank Carney, who was killed in a motor vehicle accident on June 29, 1997. The Yateses (parents of Frank) and the Cahills decided that a golf tournament would be an excellent way to raise monies for scholarships in both boys' names. Both families had been dealing with staggering grief since the deaths of their sons. The golf tournament idea was born to remember what Matt and

Frank stood for as individuals: energetic, fun-loving fellows full of the excitement of living their lives. They decided: Why not encourage everyone to remember them in such a way?

- If you have lost someone you love due to NF or are in a position to make a financial contribution, consider donations to NNFF, Strategies for LIFE, or one of the researchers mentioned in Chapter 7 of this book in lieu of flowers. For more information, see the Resources section of this book.

What Physicians Can Do to Get the Word Out

There is a tendency among the health care community to keep a case of NF "hush-hush" to avoid inciting fear in the community. In light of the rarity of the disease, this is understandable. And yet, wouldn't we be better served to utilize a sudden case of NF in the community to educate the general public? So many people have contacted us—diabetics, post-surgical patients, and parents of children who have lost limbs to a battle of post-chickenpox NF—who tell us, "I had no idea that this could happen," and "Why weren't we informed?"

While NF is uncommon, nevertheless, we believe the public should be made aware of the fact that it *could* happen—in the same way that other rare conditions are—such as toxic shock syndrome (TSS), which is often associated with tampon use, and Reye's Syndrome, correlated with aspirin use in children.

We invite physicians to join us in our efforts to save lives by educating their patients about the atypical but real threat of necrotizing soft tissue infections. This holds especially true for physicians treating higher risk groups such as diabetics, the elderly, severely immunocompromised people, and children.

Discussing Your Illness with Others

Upon returning to work or rejoining community activities, many NF survivors find themselves dealing with curiosity, fear, and misunderstanding from friends, coworkers, and even complete strangers regarding their illness. One NF survivor, a young wife and mother residing in a small seaside community in Maine, recalled shopping for groceries shortly after her release from the hospital and overhearing two women fretting for their safety because of recent news reports about a flesh-eating bacteria victim in their own town. She couldn't believe they were talking about her.

The question "Is it true you had the flesh-eating bacteria?" from a curious coworker or neighbor could invoke a growl of "Mind your own blankety-blank business!" from one NF survivor, while another may whip out the photo album or yank up his shirt to proudly display his battle scars. Another survivor may be hesitant to discuss the experience at all. How do you cope with the stares and clumsy but well-meaning questions? Moreover, how do you handle requests from the media for interviews—sometimes when the NF victim is still hospitalized? We'll offer some practical suggestions for coping with these issues in the following paragraphs.

Coping with Questions from Friends, Neighbors, and Coworkers

- Decide as a family how much information is for public knowledge, and guide your conversations and actions accordingly.
- Understand that the disease is profoundly misunderstood, and give the benefit of the doubt. Perhaps preface your answer with, "I'm not surprised you'd be under that impression. That is a common misperception. The truth is . . ."
- Offer your friends and acquaintances resources for educating themselves regarding the disease: this book, the URL of the National Necrotizing Fasciitis Foundation Web site (www.nnff.org), your doctor's telephone number, etc.
- Send thank-you notes to those who prayed for you or sent get-well cards or flowers or visited in the hospital, taking the opportunity to explain briefly that you survived a devastating illness, but despite common misperceptions, no one should fear contracting it from you.
- Upon returning to the workplace, consider speaking to concerned employees as a group to discuss your experience and to offer further

information to help everyone become aware of the disease. Provide opportunities for questions, with the caveat that no question will be considered inappropriate.

Coping with the Media

We sat together as a family in the ICU waiting room, holding each other and praying as our mother fought for her life in surgery. A nurse came over and quietly informed us that the local television station was outside doggedly requesting to interview us for the ten o'clock news. "The flesh-eating bacteria is big news," she explained. "I don't know how they found out, but they did. I'm sorry." We felt invaded upon to say the least and immediately declined. We decided if Mom would like her story to be told when and if she survived, then that would be her decision.

—"Marco"

Make no mistake about it—sometimes the media can be as vicious as the actual disease: invasive and relentless. When the story gets out about a flesh-eating bacteria victim in town, NF victims or their grieving families find themselves having to cope with television crews camped outside the hospital and repeated requests for interviews from pushy reporters—with or without the offer of financial compensation. It can be heady stuff to be thrust into the limelight under such circumstances. In the next few paragraphs we offer advice for NF victims and their families when dealing with the media:

- You have the right to privacy if you so desire. If you do not wish to have your name released, you don't have to. Instruct the public relations staff of the hospital of your wishes.
- If your loved one is unconscious, consider waiting until the patient can make the personal decision to discuss his or her experience with the media. Understandably, the stigma of being a flesh-eating bacteria victim may not be appealing to many people.

- If you do grant an interview, insist on being able to proofread print media for accuracy prior to the article's being published. Reporters can inadvertently misquote or misinterpret your responses. It is better to edit the article before it is published than to issue a tiny, seldom-noted correction afterwards. Many may not agree to this, but it is worth a try.
- Telling your story when the dust settles with a compassionate journalist can be very therapeutic to the NF victim and/or the surviving family. We've read several well-written articles that combine the courageous personal story of the victim with accurate information regarding the disease that increased awareness for the general public and even resulted in donations for the patient's medical bills.
- It almost goes without saying, but be aware that some forms of media—certain tabloids, for instance—will unscrupulously exaggerate, inflame, stretch, and twist the story you tell them, and then top it off with a ridiculous headline for the simple purpose of selling newspapers. Carefully consider the venue in which you choose to share your story: You may suddenly find yourself as the world's most famous victim of an incurable strain of flesh-eating disease that you contracted on board the spaceship of evil aliens.

It is part of our nature to panic in the face of fear and misunderstanding, particularly when it comes to a disease as swift-moving and deadly as necrotizing fasciitis. However, through our efforts to become informed about the nature of invasive infections—how they are contracted, their symptoms, and how we can protect ourselves—our fear can be greatly reduced and our actions can be guided by common sense, based on the facts. It is our greatest hope that this book has provided comprehensive information, guideposts, and sound advice to assist the reader—NF survivor, surviving relative, layperson, health care provider, teacher, or student—in understanding necrotizing fasciitis. And through this understanding, we pray that we have provided our readers with the means to empower themselves if NF should ever touch their lives.

Conclusion

⑥

WE REALIZE that people have read this book for a variety of reasons: some have had NF and survived it, while others have lost family members to it. Some may be doing research, while others may just be curious or may want to be better informed about invasive infections.

Whatever your reason, we hope you feel that the time you have invested has been well spent. NF is a very serious subject—not the stuff of warm and fuzzy bedtime reading. Indeed, what we have described about the disease throughout this book—the lightning-fast speed with which it can destroy tissue and its ability to mimic everyday minor afflictions until it's too late—may cause bad dreams in even the most stoic of souls. And the person who has survived it, or who has watched helplessly as a family member has suffered through it, knows only too well the nightmare that is necrotizing fasciitis. Your courage is an inspiration; a testament to the strength of the human spirit.

Surviving necrotizing fasciitis is an enormous challenge. In fact, there are many who do not survive it. For those who do, physical, psychological, and spiritual recovery is a long and arduous journey. Life takes on an entirely new meaning as values shift and lifestyles change. No matter what phase of the journey you are on, no matter what limbs you are missing or scars you must bear, know that you have triumphed over one of the most deadly afflictions of our time. We hope that the true accounts we have shared throughout this book have helped you realize that you are not alone.

We salute the researchers and physicians whom we have introduced in this book, and also those unmentioned, for their tireless commitment to the ongoing battle against NF and invasive group A strep infections. We hope that you share our excitement about the emerging diagnostic tools, treatments, and vaccines that may one day make NF a thing of the past. But until then, mainstream awareness of NF—its symptoms, manifestations, treatment, and risk factors—is the most powerful weapon we have. We ask that each person who reads this book tell someone else about it. Educate someone else about NF. It may save a life one day.

Glossary

Acute. When describing an illness, one that is short-term with no recurrence, such as chicken pox.

Adult respiratory syndrome (ARS). Life-threatening complication of toxic shock characterized by fluid-filled lungs and difficulty breathing.

Aerobic. Describes bacteria that require oxygen to survive.

Amputation. The surgical removal of a limb due to disease or injury.

Anaerobic. Describes bacteria that do not require oxygen to survive.

Antibiotic. Drug that kills bacteria, thus combating infection.

Antibiotic prophylaxis. The administration of antibiotics to help fortify the body against the possibility of infection.

Antibiotic-resistant bacteria. Bacteria that have evolved to withstand antibiotics.

Bacteroides. Anaerobic bacteria found in the intestines of human beings.

Bullae. Large blisters filled with a bloody or yellowish fluid appearing on the body of an NF patient.

Cellulitis. Skin and soft-tissue infection caused by invasive Group A strep characterized by fever, mild swelling, and redness. Typically responds to antibiotics and moist heat.

Chronic. When describing an illness, long-term, perhaps worsening over time and/or frequently recurring (such as diabetes mellitus).

Clostridium. Anaerobic bacterium found in soil and the intestinal tract of some humans and animals. Associated with gas gangrene, it is a rapidly fatal form of necrotizing soft-tissue infection.

Cluster. When referring to group A strep infections, an apparent mini-outbreak of cases of invasive group A strep disease, which may or may not include necrotizing fasciitis, in a specific geographical area.

Computerized tomography (CT) scan. Imaging study that consists of a highly sensitive X-ray beam that allows a cross-section view of the inside of the body.

Debridement. Surgery to remove necrotic tissue.

Epidemic. An outbreak of disease among a population.

Exploratory surgery. Surgery performed with the intention of confirming or assisting in making a diagnosis.

Fasciae. Sheets of connective tissue surrounding muscles.

Flesh-eating bacteria. Nickname given to group A strepbacteria that cause rapidly spreading necrotizing fasciitis.

Frozen-tissue biopsy. Diagnostic tool in which a scoop or "punch" of skin is removed from a patient under local anesthesia and examined immediately for an underlying disease process.

Gangrene. Tissue death caused by disease or injury.

HEPA filter. High-efficiency particulate arresting filter. A device that reportedly removes over 98 percent of bacteria, pollen, mold spores, animal hair and dander, dust, and other airborne particles from the air.

Higher-risk groups. In terms of NF, those individuals with underlying conditions who appear to be at higher risk for contracting the disease, such as diabetics and severely immunocompromised individuals.

Hyperbaric oxygen chamber. An enclosed cylinder for medical treatment that provides 100-percent pure oxygen.

Hypotension. Low blood pressure.

ICU psychosis. Complication of long-term hospital confinement and drug therapy in which the patient experiences hallucinations.

Immunocompromised. Describes an individual whose immune system is less than adequate to defend the host from infections, due to illness, the taking of medication, etc.

Immunosuppression. The deliberate suppression of a person's immune system for medical reasons, such as his or her undergoing organ transplantation or chemotherapy.

Infectious disease. An illness that is spread from person to person.

Intravenous immunoglobulin. Sterile solution of plasma proteins harvested from a vast pool of human donations. Used to fight infection.

Invasive group A strep. A group of bacteria that penetrate the body through the blood, lungs, or openings in the skin, causing severe and life-threatening illness.

Loxosceles reclusa. The brown recluse spider, whose bite can cause a necrotic ulcer sometimes confused with NF.

Lymphedema. Condition in which damage to the lymphatic system results in chronic limb swelling, scar tissue development, and infections.

Magnetic resonance imaging (MRI). Diagnostic imaging tool that uses radio waves and huge magnets to create an intensely strong magnetic field, allowing a three-dimensional view of the inside of the body.

Malaise. General feeling of being unwell.

Meningitis. Infection of the brain and spinal cord caused by invasive group A strep bacteria.

Murcomycosis. Airborne, highly fatal infection rarely affecting human beings caused by various fungi of the *Murcales* genus, which is found in bread and fruit mold.

Necrotizing cellulitis. Progressing infection that confines itself to the subcutaneous fat, sparing the deep fascia. Sometimes a complication of untreated or inadequately treated cellulitis.

Necrotizing fascitiis/streptococcal toxic shock syndrome. Rapidly progressing, highly fatal disease most often caused by group A streptococci that causes necrosis, massive organ failure, and death.

Nosocomial infection. An infection acquired in the hospital.

Oliguria. Lack of urine output.

Organ failure. The shutdown of major internal organs such as kidneys, lungs, and heart in response to disease process.

Pathogen. A disease-causing organism, such as group A strep.

Personal air purifier. Beeper-sized device worn around the neck or in the shirt pocket that purifies air through ionization and redirects that air toward the wearer to be inhaled.

Pharyngitis. Infection of the back of the mouth or tonsils.

Pneumonia. Infection of the lungs that is caused by invasive group A strep.

Post-streptococcal glomerulonephritis. A serious affliction of the kidneys that can occur ten to fourteen days after a streptococcal infection.

Prevotella. Genus of anaerobic bacteria that can exist in the mouth and urinary and respiratory tracts. It is associated with NF that involves the face, mouth, jaw, and neck.

Prosthetics. Artificial limbs, fingers, and other body structures used to replace amputated counterparts.

Pseudomonas. Genus of bacteria associated with NF in severely immunocompromised individuals.

Pyoderma. Infection of the skin.

Reconstructive surgery. Surgery performed generally by a plastic surgeon to repair defects or to improve the appearance of scars.

Rheumatic fever. Complication of a group A strep infection that causes widespread inflammation.

Self-acquired NF. NF caused by bacteria residing in or on the patient's own body.

Septicemia. Infection of the blood caused by invasive group A strep.

Skin flaps. Full-thickness sections of skin and soft tissue used to repair defects or gaping wounds.

Skin grafting. Harvesting viable, healthy skin from one part of the body to be used on another to cover defects or gaping wounds.

Spontaneous NF infections. NF infections that have no evident point of entry.

Staphylococcus aureus. Aerobic bacteria often involved in NF in conjunction with other types of bacteria. Also causes a variety of other conditions including boils and food poisoning.

Sepsis. Toxicity due to a bacterial infection.

Serotype. Variation of a particular type of bacteria.

Strep throat. Infection of the throat and tonsils caused by group A strep bacteria.

Subcutaneous tissue. Soft tissue located beneath the skin and above the muscles.

Systemic toxicity. Condition in which toxins are traveling throughout the body.

Tachycardia. Rapid and shallow heartbeat.

Tachypnea. Rapid breathing.

Tissue expansion. Stretching of skin using a balloon-type apparatus to repair defects or gaping wounds.

Toxic shock. State in which toxins flooding a patient's body due to a disease process cause the body to go into shock.

Undermining. When referring to NF, the separation of the soft tissue from the fasciae.

Vacuum-assisted closure. Type of vacuum that utilizes negative pressure to aid in wound closure and the removal of fluids that can impede healing.

Vibrio vulnificus. Bacterium that occurs naturally in estuarine waters and resides in high numbers in filter-feeding shellfish such as oysters, clams, and mussels.

Resources

❦

Amputation

Books

Challenged by Amputation: Embracing a New Life, Carol S. Wallace, M.S., CRC, Inclusion Concepts Publishing House, 1995

Organizations

American Amputee Foundation, Inc. (AAF)
PO Box 250218
Hillcrest Station
Little Rock, Arkansas 72225
(501)666-2523
Fax: (501)666-8367

Emotional Freedom Techniques/ Trauma Incident Reduction

Emotional Freedom Techniques™
Gary H. Craig
PO Box 398, The Sea Ranch, CA 95497

(707)785-2848
www.emofree.com

Deborah Mitnick, LCSW-C
Specialized Treatment for Rapid Emotional Healing, Personal
    Performance Coaching, Trauma Relief Services
6525 North Charles Street
Gibson Building, Suite 042
Towson, MD 21204
(410)494-1002
fax (410)385-5770
dmitnick@qis.net
www.trauma-tir.com

Group A Strep Surveillance

Centers for Disease Control and Prevention (CDC)
Division of Bacterial and Mycotic Diseases
Active Bacterial Core Surveillance
1600 Clifton Road
MS A-49
Atlanta GA 30333
www.cdc.gov/ncidod/dbmd/abcs/default.htm

Ontario Group A Streptococcal Study
Department of Microbiology, Mount Sinai Hospital
600 University Avenue, Room 1460
Toronto, Ontario, Canada, M5G 1X5
Donald Low, MD, Microbiologist-in-Chief / Infectious Diseases
Allison McGeer, MD, Microbiologist / Infectious Diseases / Infection
    Control
(800)668-6292

Holistic Counseling

Irene Koenig, Certified Pathwork
Helper, Teacher, Core Energetics
65 Prospect Avenue
Niantic, CT 06357
(860)739-6865

fax (860)739-5782
www.holisticcounseling.org
thepathik@aol.com
*Counseling for the whole person—body, mind, spirit; practical healing for the
soul. Offered in person or via telephone or written correspondence.*

Necrotizing Fasciitis/Group A Strep Organizations

The Lee Spark NF Foundation
Severe Streptococcal Infections and Necrotizing Fasciitis Support
Telephone/fax 012-487-8701
cmarsden@zen.co.uk

The National Necrotizing Fasciitis Foundation
2731 Porter SW
Grand Rapids, MI 49509

25 Prospect Avenue
Niantic, CT 06357

Toll free (888)550-NNFF
www.nnff.org

Surviving Strep—Strategies for LIFE
(905)257-0007
www.dynamite@cgo cable.net
www.cgocable.net/~lifehike

Necrotizing Fasciitis/Group A Strep Books

Miracle Victory over the Flesh-Eating Bacteria by David L. Cowles and
Delys Cowles, Gibbs Smith Publishers, 1997
*Streptococcal Infections: Clinical Aspects, Microbiology, and Molecular Patho-
genesis,* edited by Dennis L. Stevens and Edward L. Kaplan, Ox-
ford, 1999

Plastic and Reconstructive Surgery

Foundation for Plastic and Reconstruction Surgery
(212)794-1234
www.frps.org

American Society of Plastic Surgeons (ASPS) and the Plastic Surgery
   Educational Foundation (PSEF).
444 E. Algonquin Road
Arlington Heights, IL 60005
(888)4-PLASTIC

Researchers, Group A Strep Vaccines

James B. Dale, M.D.
Professor of Medicine
Chief, Division of Infectious Diseases
The University of Tennessee and VA Medical Center
1030 Jefferson Avenue
Memphis, TN 38104

Vincent A. Fischetti, Ph.D.
Rockefeller University
1230 York Avenue
New York, NY 10021
www.rockefeller.edu/vaf

Prosthetics

Aesthetic Concerns
Two Edge Water Drive, Suite 201
Middletown, NY 10940
(800)208-SKIN
Fax (914)344-6829

Alatheia Prosthetic Rehabilitation Center
504 Grants Ferry Road
Brandon, MS 39047

(877) ALATHEIA
E-mail: info@alatheia.org
www.alatheia.org

Support and Information
Orthotics & Prosthetics Online Community
www.oandp.com
(comprehensive Web site including directory of product suppliers, patient-care
    facilities, organizations and associations, news, support, etc.)

U.S. Government Agencies
Centers for Disease Control and Prevention (CDC)
1600 Clifton Road
Atlanta, GA 30333
USA
(800)311-3435
www.cdc.gov

National Institutes of Health (NIH)
Bethesda, MD 20892
(800)411-1222
www.nih.gov

Vibrio Valnificus
James D. Oliver
Cone Distinguished Professor
Professor of Microbiology and Director, Interdisciplinary
    Biotechnology Program
University of North Carolina at Charlotte
9201 University City Boulevard
Charlotte, NC 28223-0001
(704)547-4049
Fax (704)547-3457

www.vibrio.com
E-mail: jdoliver@email.uncc.edu

Wound Care

The Wound Care Institute
1100 NE 163rd Street, Suite 101
North Miami Beach, FL 33162
www.woundcare.org

References

❦

1. *What Is Necrotizing Fasciitis?*

Barillo, D. J. "Dermatologists and the Burn Center." *Dermatol Clin* 17 (1) (1999):61–75, viii.

Bisno, A. L., and D. L. Stevens. "Streptococcal Infections of Skin and Soft Tissues." *N Engl J Med* 334 (1996):240–245.

Bollet, A. J. "Necrotizing Fascitis: Return of a Major Civil War Disease." *Infectious Disease Historical Vignette* (1997):4.

Bollet, J. Alfred, M.D., Yale University School of Medicine. Personal Communication. June 30, 1998

Brogan, T. V., and V. Nizet. "A Clinical Approach to Differentiating Necrotizing Fasciitis From Simple Cellulitis." *Infections in Medicine* 14(9) (1997):734–738.

Campbell, J. R. "An Outbreak of M Serotype 1 Group A Streptococcus in a Neonatal Intensive Care Unit." *J Pediatr* 129(3) (1996):396–402.

Chapnick, E. K., and E. I. Abter. "Infectious Disease Emergencies, Necrotizing Soft-Tissue Infections." *Infectious Disease Clinics of North America* 10(4) (1996):835–850.

Condon, R. E. and Rakel. "Necrotizing Skin and Soft Tissue Infections." *Conn's Current Therapy,* 50th ed. (1998):87–89.

Grant, A. "Streptococcus A—Necrotizing Fascitis." Emergency.com, June 18, 1997, www.emergency.com/strep-a.htm

Green, R. J., D. C. Dafoe, and T. A. Raffin. "Necrotizing Fasciitis." *Chest* 110 (1) (1996):220–230.

Hill, M. K. "Skin and Soft Tissue Infections in Critical Care." *Crit Care Clin* 14(2) (1998):251–262.

Illinois Dept of Public Health, "Group A Streptococcus." *IL Dept of Public Health Healthbeat* (1997).

Morse, S. S. "Factors in the Emergence of Infectious Diseases." *EID* 1 (1) (1999).

Musher, D. M., et al. "Trends in Bacteremic Infection Due to Streptococcus pyogenes (Group A Streptococcus), 1986–1995." *Emerging Infectious Diseases* 2(1) (1996):54–56.

Reese, R. E. "Necrotizing Soft-Tissue Infections." *Practical Approach to Infectious Diseases,* 4th ed. (1996):114–117.

Rosen, P. "Cellulitis." *Emergency Medicine: Concepts and Clinical Practice,* 4th ed. (1998):2670–2672.

Stevens, D. L. "The Toxic Shock Syndromes." *Infect Dis Clin North Am* 10(4) (1996):727–746.

Valentine, E. G. "Nontraumatic Gas Gangrene." *Ann Emerg Med* 30(1) (1997):109–111.

Weiss, R. "Virulent Outbreak of Strep Hits Texas." *Washington Post* (1998):A03

Wilson, A. "Disease Claims Man's Fingers, Toes." *The Salt Lake Tribune* (1997).

Wilson, B. "Necrotizing Fasciitis." *Am Surg* 18 (1952):416–431

"Research on Microbial Changes and Adaptations Influencing Emergence." www.niaid.nih.gov/publications/execsum/1a.htm

"Group A Streptococcus." www.cdc.gov, January 1, 1999, www.cdc.gov/ncidod/diseases/bacter/strep_a.htm

"Necrotizing Fasciitis." www.meded.uci.edu/-surgery/handout6.html

2. *How NF Is Contracted*

Anderson, P. C. "Spider Bites in the United States." *Dermatol Clin* 15(2) (1997):307–311.

Barillo, D. J. "Dermatologists and the Burn Center." *Dermatol Clin* 17(1) (1999):61–75, viii.

Bisno, A. L., and D. L. Stevens. "Streptococcal Infections of Skin and Soft Tissues." *N Engl J Med* 334 (1996):240–245.

Bollet, J. Alfred, M.D., Yale University School of Medicine. Personal Communication. January 4, 1998.

Brogan, T. V., and V. Nizet. "A Clinical Approach to Differentiating Necrotizing Fasciitis from Simple Cellulitis." *Infections in Medicine* 14(9) (1997):734–738.

Childs, S. G. "Necrotizing Fasciitis: Challenging Management of a Septic Wound." *Orthopaedic Nursing* (1999):11–19.

Condon, R. E. and Rakel. "Necrotizing Skin and Soft Tissue Infections." *Conn's Current Therapy,* 50th ed. (1998):87–89.

Dale, James, M.D. Personal Communication, March, 1999.

Giitter, M. "Adjunctive Hyperbaric Oxygen Therapy in the Treatment of Rhinocerebral Mucormycosis." *Infect Med 2* (1996):130–136.

Lemonick, M.D. "Streptomania Hits Home, A Bacterial Strain That Terrified Britain Pops Up in the U.S., but Doctors Say There's No Need to Panic." *Time Domestic* 143(25) (1994).

McHenry, Christopher R., et al. "Determinants of Mortality for NSTI." *Annals of Surgery* 221(5) (1995)

Morrison, G. W. "A Long Journey Home." *Flair. The Grand Rapids Press* (1998):C1–C2.

Nomikos, I. N. "Necrotizing Perineal Infections (Fournier's Disease): Old Remedies for an Old Disease." *Int J Colorectal Dis* 13(1) (1998): 48–51.

Ramage, L., et al. *Infect Control Hosp Epidemiol* 17 (1996):429–431.

Reuters. "Hospital Infections on the Rise." www.abcnews.com

Schreuder, F., and M. Chatoo. "Another Cause of Necrotizing Fasciitis." *J Infect* 35(2) (1997):177–178.

Species 2000, www.sp2000.org June 18, 2000

Stevens, D. L. "Streptococcal Toxic-Shock Syndrome: Spectrum of Disease, Pathogenesis, and New Concepts in Treatment." *EID* 1(3) (1995).

State of Texas Department of Health, www.tdh.texas.gov/phpep/strepa.htm

Weinstein, R. A. "Nosocomial Infection Update." *Emerging Infectious Diseases.* Vol. 4 No. 3 (July–Sept 1998): 416–419.

Wilson, A. " Disease Eats Mans Fingers and Toes." *The Salt Lake Tribune* (1996):B1.

Wright, S. W. "Clinical Presentation and Outcome of Brown Recluse Spider Bite." *Ann Emerg Med* 30(1) (1997):28–32.

"Research on Microbial Changes and Adaptations Influencing Emergence." www.niaid.nih.gov/publications/execsum/1 a.htm

"The Worldwide Intensivist," www.anaesthetist.com/icu/infect/fungi/mucor.htm

"Vibrio vulnificus homepage." www.vibrio.com

3. *Opportunities for Infection and Higher-Risk Groups*

AAP. "Infection Control for Hospitalized Children." *AAP 1997 Red Book: Report of The Committee on Infectious Diseases,* 24th ed. (1997):100–107.

American Diabetes Association. www.diabetes.org, February 1999.

American Obesity Association. www.obesity.org, February, 1999.

Baker, B. "Ibuprofen Tied to Necrotizing Fasciitis in Varicella." *Pediatric News* 31(11) (1997):32.

Balch, J., and P. Balch. *Prescription for Nutritional Healing,* 2nd ed. (1997):241.

Bisno, A. L., and D. L. Stevens. "Streptococcal Infections of Skin and Soft Tissues." *N Engl J Med* 334 (1996):240–245

Campbell, J. R. "An Outbreak of M Serotype 1 Group A Streptococcus in a Neonatal Intensive Care Unit." *J Pediatr* 129(3) (1996):396–402.

Chapnick, E. K., and E. I. Abter. "Infectious Disease Emergencies, Necrotizing Soft-Tissue Infections." *Infectious Disease Clinics of North America* 10(4) (1996):835–850.

Christensen, D. "Elderly at Risk of Contracting 'Flesh-Eating' Bacteria." *The New England Journal of Medicine* 335 (1996):547–554.

Davies, H. D., et al. "Invasive Group A Streptococcal Infections in Ontario, Canada." *The New England Journal of Medicine* 335(8) (1996).

EID. "CDC Convenes Meeting to Discuss Strategies for Preventing Invasive Group A Streptococcal Infectious." *EID* 2(1) (1996).

Elliott, D. C., et al. "Necrotizing Soft Tissue Infections, Risk Factors for Mortality and Strategies for Management." *Annals of Surgery* 224(5) (1996):673–680.

Estrada, B. "Varicella and GAS: Do NSAIDs Fuel the Fire?" *Infections in Medicine* 16(5) (1999):307.

Halsey, N. A., et al. "Severe Invasive Group A Streptococcal Infections: A Subject Review." *Pediatrics* 101(1) (1998):136–139.

Holder, E. P., P. T. Moore, and B. A. Browne. "Nonsteroidal Anti-Inflammatory Drugs and Necrotising Fasciitis. An Update." *Drug Saf* 17(6) (1997):369–373.

Kahn, L. H., and B. A. Styrt. "Necrotizing Soft Tissue Infections Reported with Nonsteroidal Anti-Inflammatory Drugs." *Annals of Pharmacotherapy* 31(9) (1997):1034–1039.

Lede, R., et al. "Is routine use of episiotomy justified?" *American Journal of Obstetrics and Gynecology* 175(5) (1996):1399–1402.

McHenry, Christopher R., et al. "Determinants of Mortality for NSTI." *Annals of Surgery* 221(5) (1995).

Michalsen, A., et al. "Compliance with Universal Precautions Among Physicians." *Journal of Occupational and Environmental Medicine* 39(2) (1997):130–137.

Myers-Helfgott, M. G. "Routine Use of Episiotomy in Modern Obstetrics. Should It Be performed?" *Obstet Gynecol Clin North Am* 26(2) (1999):305–325.

Reese, R. E. "General Principles of Wound Infection Management." *Practical Approach to Infectious Diseases,* 4th ed. (1996):122–125.

Reese, R. E. "Necrotizing Soft-Tissue Infections." *Practical Approach to Infectious Diseases,* 4th ed. (1996):114–117.

Rosen, P. "Cellulitis." *Emergency Medicine: Concepts and Clinical Practice,* 4th ed. (1998):2670–2672.

Zerr, D. M. "A Case-Control Study of Necrotizing Fasciitis during Primary Varicella." *Pediatrics* 103(4) Pt. 1 (1999):783–790.

Zurawski, C. A., et al. "Invasive Group A Streptococcal Disease in Metropolitan Atlanta: A Population-Based Assessment." *Clin Infect Dis* 27(1) (1998):150–157.

"Deadly Viruses, The Virus-Bacteria Double Whammy." *Redbook* (1997).

4: *Making the Diagnosis*

Barillo, D. J. "Dermatologists and the Burn Center." *Dermatol Clin* 17(1) (1999):61–75, viii.

Bilton, B. D., et al. "Aggressive Surgical Management of Necrotizing Fasciitis Serves to Decrease Mortality: a Retrospective Study." *American Surgeon* 64(5) (1998):397–400.

Brogan, T. V., and V. Nizet. "A Clinical Approach to Differentiating Necrotizing Fasciitis from Simple Cellulitis." *Infections in Medicine* 14(9) (1997):734–738.

Chao, H. C., M. S. Kong, and T. Y. Lin. "Diagnosis of Necrotizing Fasciitis in Children." *Journal of Ultrasound in Medicine* 18(4) (1999):277–281.

Chapnick, E. K., and E. I. Abter. "Infectious Disease Emergencies, Necrotizing Soft-Tissue Infections." *Infectious Disease Clinics of North America* 10(4) (1996):835–850.

Childs, S. G. "Necrotizing Fasciitis: Challenging Management of a Septic Wound." *Orthopaedic Nursing* (1999):11–19.

Condon, R. E. and Rakel. "Necrotizing Skin and Soft Tissue Infections." *Conn's Current Therapy,* 50th ed. (1998):87–89.

Elliott, D. C., et al. "Necrotizing Soft Tissue Infections, Risk Factors for Mortality and Strategies for Management." *Annals of Surgery* 224(5) (1996):673–680.

File, T. M., Jr., J. S. Tan, and J. R. DiPersio. "Group A Streptococcal Necrotizing Fasciitis. Diagnosing and Treating the 'Flesh-Eating Bacteria Syndrome.' " *Cleve Clin J Med* 65(5) (1998):241–249.

Green, R. J., D. C. Dafoe, and T. A. Raffin. "Necrotizing Fasciitis." *Chest* 110(1) (1996):220–23.

Hollands, L. S. "Part 1 Necrotizing Fasciitis: Diagnosis." *British Columbia Medical Journal* 41(4) (1999):172–173.

Hollands, L. S. "Necrotizing Fasciitis: An Approach to Initial Diagnosis and Empiric Management." *British Columbia Medical Journal* 41(4) (1999):174–176.

Kujath, P. "Correspondence." *N Engl J Med* 336 (1997):513–514.

Leong, W. C., et al. "Severe Soft-Tissue Infections—a Diagnostic Challenge. The Need for Early Recognition and Aggressive Therapy." *S Afr Med J* 87(5 Suppl) (1997):648–652, 654.

McHenry, Christopher R., et al. "Determinants of Mortality for NSTI." *Annals of Surgery* 221(5) (1995).

Reese, R. E. "Necrotizing Soft-Tissue Infections." *Practical Approach to Infectious Diseases,* 4th ed. (1996):114–117.

Rosen, P. "Cellulitis." *Emergency Medicine: Concepts and Clinical Practice,* 4th ed. (1998):2670–2672.

Scher, R. L. "Hyperbaric Oxygen Therapy for Necrotizing Cervical Infections." *Adv Otorhinolaryngol* 54 (1998):50–58.

Stevens, D. L. "Necrotizing Fasciitis: Don't Wait to Make a Diagnosis." *Infect Med* 14(9) (1997):684, 688.

Stevens, D. L. "Streptococcal Toxic-Shock Syndrome: Spectrum of Disease, Pathogenesis, and New Concepts in Treatment." *EID* 1(3) (1995).

Stone, D. R., and S. L. Gorbach. "Necrotizing Fasciitis. The Changing Spectrum." *Dermatol Clin* 15(2) (1997):213–220.

"Group A Streptococcus." www.cdc.gov, www.cdc.gov/ncidod/diseases/bacter/strep_a.htm

"Necrotizing Fasciitis." www.meded.uci.edu/~surgery/handout6.html

5: *Why NF Is Often Misdiagnosed*

Brisno, Alan, personal communication, June 1999.

Brogan, T. V., and V. Nizet. "A Clinical Approach to Differentiating Necrotizing Fasciitis from Simple Cellulitis." *Infections in Medicine* 14(9) (1997):734–738.

Collins, K. S., et al. "Resource for HMO Information." *The Commonwealth Fund Survey of Physician Experiences with Managed Care* (1997).

Condon, R. E. and Rakel. "Necrotizing Skin and Soft Tissue Infections." *Conn's Current Therapy,* 50th ed. (1998):87–89.

Green, R. J., D. C. Dafoe, and T. A. Raffin. "Necrotizing Fasciitis." *Chest* 110(1) (1996):220–230.

Hollands, L. S. "Part 1 Necrotizing Fasciitis: Diagnosis." *British Columbia Medical Journal* 41(4) (1999):172–173.

Hollands, L. S. "Necrotizing Fasciitis: An Approach to Initial Diagnosis and Empiric Management." *British Columbia Medical Journal* 41(4) (1999):174–176.

Hollands, Laurence, personal communication, June 2000.

McHenry, Christopher R., et al. "Determinants of Mortality for NSTI." *Annals of Surgery* 221(5) (1995).

Reese, R. E. "Necrotizing Soft-Tissue Infections." *Practical Approach to Infectious Diseases,* 4th ed. (1996):114–117.

Rivey, M. P., D. R. Allington, and A. L. Henry Durham. "Necrotizing Fasciitis Associated with Nonsteroidal Antiinflammatory Drug Use." *J Pharm Technol* 14 (1998):58–62.

Rosen. "Cellulitis." *Emergency Medicine: Concepts and Clinical Practice,* 4th ed. (1998):2670–2672.

Stevens, D. L. "Necrotizing Fasciitis: Don't Wait to Make a Diagnosis" *Infect Med* 14(9) (1997):684, 688.

Stevens, Dennis, personal communication, March 1999.

Triesenberg, Steven, personal communication, April 2000.

Vugia, D. J., et al. "Outbreak of Invasive Group A Streptococcus Associated with Varicella in a Childcare Center—Boston, Massachusetts, 1997." *Pediatric Infect Dis J* 15 (1996):146–150.

6. *Treatment of NF*

Barillo, D. J. "Dermatologists and the Burn Center." *Dermatol Clin* 17(1) (1999):61–75, viii.

Bisno, Alan L., personal communication, June 2000.

Cranton, E. M. "Hyperbaric Oxygen." *Bypassing Bypass* (1998).

Childs, S. G. "Necrotizing Fasciitis: Challenging Management of a Septic Wound." *Orthopaedic Nursing* (1999):11–19.

Green, R. J., D. C. Dafoe, and T. A. Raffin. "Necrotizing Fasciitis." *Chest* 110(1) (1996):220–230.

Hammond, Dennis, plastic surgeon, Grand Rapids, MI, personal communication, October 1999.

Hollands, L. S. "Part 1 Necrotizing Fasciitis: Diagnosis." *British Columbia Medical Journal* 41(4) (1999):172–173.

Low, Donald, personal communication, March 1999.

McGinn, Kerry, and Haylock, Pamela, "Muscle Flap Reconstructive Procedures." WebMD.com, April 9, 2000, www.my.webmd.com/content/dmk/dmk_article_3961071

McHenry, Christopher, personal communication, March 1999.

Mosher, M. C. "Surgical Management of Necrotizing Fasciitis." *British Columbia Medical Journal* 41(5) (1999):220–224.

Stevens, Dennis L., personal communication, March 1999.

Triesenberg, N. Steven, M.D., Infectious Diseases Specialist. Personal communication. April 26, 2000.

Triesenberg, Steven, personal communication, April 2000.

West, Carolyn, and John T. Mather Memorial Hospital Hyperbaric Oxygen Unit, Personal communication, April 1998.

"Skin Grafts." Medical OnLine.com, April 9, 2000, www.medicalonline.com.au/medical/disease_index/plastic_surgery/grafts.htm

"Skin Graft." Healthgate.com, April 9, 2000, www.healthgate.com/sym/surg139.shtml,

"Skin Graft." HealthCentral.com, General Health Encyclopedia, April 9, 2000, www,healthcentral.com/mhc/top/002982.cfm

"Skin Graft." WebMD.com, powered by adam.com, April 9, 2000, my.webmd.com/content/asset/adam_surgery_skin_graft

7. *Emerging Treatments*

Abraham, C. "Antibody Cocktail Cheats Flesh-Eating Disease." *The Globe and Mail* (1999).

Bisno, Alan L., personal communication, June 1999.

Congkit, Rene, et al., "The Use of Capsular Reactive Protein (CRP) for the Dectection and Monitoring of Serious Infections and Gross Soft Tissue Necrosis." *British Columbia Medical Journal* 41(4) (1999):177–179.

Dale, J. B. "Group A Streptoccal Vaccines." *Infect Dis Clin North Am* 13(1)(1999):227–43, viii.

Dale, James, personal communication, July 1999.

Habib, M. "Flesh-Eating Disease: Old Therapy Becomes New Again." *Montreal Gazette* (1999).

Holler, Anthony, ID Biomedical, personal communication, March 2000.

Kaul R., et al. "Intravenous Immunoglobulin Therapy for Streptococcal Toxic Shock Syndrome—a Comparative Observational Study, The Canadian Streptococcal Study Group." *Clinical Infectious Diseases* 28(4) (1999):800–7.

Low, Donald, personal communication, March 1999.

Majeski, J. "Necrotizing Fasciitis: Improved Survival with Early Recognition by Tissue Biopsy and Aggressive Surgical Treatment." *South Med J* 90(11) (1997):1065–1068.

Morrow, K. J. "Potential Therapeutic Attack Points for Aggressive Group A Strep Infections." *Genetic Engineering News* (1994).

Papp, L. "Toronto Study Strikes Blow against Flesh-Eating Disease." *The Toronto Star* A10 (1999).

Robinson, George, Pathologist. Personal Communication. March 25, 1999.

Zaret, B. L. *Yale University School of Medicine Patient's Guide to Medical Tests.*

9. *Continuing the Recovery Process after Hospitalization*

Cohen, Alan, personal communication, February 2000.

Fishman, Tamara, The Wound Care Institute, North Miami, FL, personal communication, April 2000.

Harrison, Mitzi, personal communication, May 30, 2000.

Keiser, Lana (Registered Occupational Therapist and Certified Hand Therapist), and Shelly Davis, of Novacare, Grand Rapids, Michigan, personal communication, June 11, 2000.

Wallace, Carol S., personal communication, May 20, 2000.

Wallace, Carol S., M.S. *Challenged by Amputation: Embracing a New Life,* CRC. Fair Oaks, CA: Inclusion Concepts Publishing House, 1995.

www.apta.org (American Physical Therapy Association)

10. *Psychological, Emotional, and Spiritual Recovery*

Beers, Mark H., M.D., and Robert Berkow, M.D. *The Merck Manual of Diagnosis and Therapy,* Section 15, Chapter 189 Mood Disorders. White House Station, NJ: Merck and Co., 1999.

Balch, J. *Prescription for Nutritional Healing,* 2 ed. Garden City Park, NY: Avery Publishing Group, 1997, 241.

Earley, Jay, personal communication, March 1999.

Koenig, Irene, personal communication, June 1999.

Mitnick, Deborah, personal communication, March 1999.

Naturopathic Medicine Network, www.pandamedicine.com, May 20, 2000.

Wallace, Carol S., M.S. *Challenged by Amputation: Embracing a New Life,* CRC. Fair Oaks, CA: Inclusion Concepts Publishing House, 1995.

www.botanical.com, September, 1999.

www.healthcentral.com, September, 1999.

www.prozac.com, November 1999.

www.wellbrutrin.com, November 1999.

11. *Awareness and Prevention: What You Can Do*

American Academy of Pediactrics, www.aap.org, April, 1999.

Complete Guide to Symptoms, Illness and Surgery, 2d ed. Los Angeles: The Body Press/Perigee, 1989, 542.

Bisno, A. L. Diagnosis and Management of Group A Streptococcal Pharyngitis: a Practice Guideline. Presented at the Infectious Diseases Society of America 35th Annual Meeting. Sept. 13–16, 1997, San Francisco.

Additional References

The World Health Organization Liaison Office in Washington (WDC), 1775 K Street NW, Suite 430, Washington, D.C. 20006.

Index

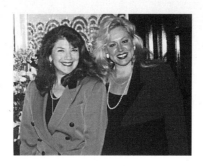

ABOUT THE AUTHORS

Jacqueline Roemmele is a professional multimedia consultant and website developer, as well as a freelance writer. She was stricken with necrotizing fasciitis in 1993 after suffering from an undiagnosed postoperative infection. She lives in Connecticut with her husband, Rick, and her three sons, Vincent, Alex, and Ricardo.

Donna Batdorff is an advertising salesperson for a cable television company. Her bout with necrotizing fasciitis followed a small cut she suffered on her finger while skiing in 1996. She lives in Grand Rapids, Michigan. The authors found each other through the Internet, and in 1997 founded the National Necrotizing Fasciitis Foundation.